Women and Health

THE MAGILL BIBLIOGRAPHIES

Women and Health

An Annotated Bibliography

Frances R. Belmonte

Magill Bibliographies

The Scarecrow Press, Inc.
Lanham, Md., & London
and
Salem Press
Pasadena, Calif., & Englewood Cliffs, N.J.
1997

SCARECROW PRESS, INC.

Published in the United States of America
by Scarecrow Press, Inc.
4720 Boston Way
Lanham, Maryland 20706

4 Pleydell Gardens, Folkestone
Kent CT20 2DN, England

British Library Cataloguing in Publication Information Available

Library of Congress Cataloging-in-Publication Data

Belmonte, Frances R.
    Women and health : an annotated bibliography / Frances R. Belmonte.
       p. cm. — (Magill bibliographies)
    Includes index.
    ISBN 0-8108-3385-9 (cloth : alk. paper)
    1. Women—Health and hygiene—Bibliography. I. Title. II. Series.
Z6671.845   1997
[RA564.85]
016.613'04244—dc21   97-22482
                                                 CIP

ISBN 0-8108-3385-9 (cloth : alk. paper)

The paper used in this publication meets the minimum requirements of American National Standard for Information Sciences—Permanence of Paper for Printed Library Materials, ANSI Z39.48–1984.
Manufactured in the United States of America.

This book is dedicated to Michaelle E. Bamberger and to all women
whose life work is concerned with healing.

CONTENTS

ACKNOWLEDGMENTS

To Howard Lintz, Patti Huiras and Larry Huiras whose computer assistance brought this work to closure, to Joya D'Cruz and Mary Petzel whose library assistance was invaluable, and to Michaelle Bamberger, the friend who provided personal encouragement, patience and support, I express gratitude.

INTRODUCTION

In recent years the concerns of women's health as a professional expertise, and concerns about women's health as a personal and societal issue, have come more clearly to the attention of the general public. Changes in views of women, in medical science, in history, in religion, and in psychology, have raised interconnected questions in the human community and in the healing professions. It is particularly appropriate, now that the Women's Health Movement has seen thirty years of growth, that one gather in bibliographic form some considerations specific to women and health. Particularly timely, now that the Boston Women's Health Book Collective has seen its twenty-fifth anniversary, this book encourages its readers to two activities: first, to ask the larger questions behind individual medical discoveries and procedures; and second, to see an integrated picture of women's whole health across the lifespan. While concrete scientific information changes quickly and some data may well be on its way to obsolescence even as we speak, the history, philosophy, and sociology which underlie the changes have taken centuries to move. It is thus appropriate that there be background considerations in each section. This book seeks to gather in one place pertinent considerations around the questions and bibliographic data addressing multiple facets of women and health, and insights pertinent to these considerations. The book is divided into topical sections, each interconnected with the others. These topical relationships stem from notions more akin to quantum interconnected approaches than Newtonian cause/effect ones, more akin to "women's ways of knowing" types of epistemologies than mutually exclusive logical categories, and more akin to very old "mutually indwelling" notions of Christian theology. Thus, the annotations under each topic, while not logically separate from those under the other topics, have a different accent. It is well-nigh impossible,

1

given the epistemology and the history involved, to definitively separate honoring women's health from honoring the healing professions vis-à-vis women, from honoring women's caring for from honoring women's being cared for. The wholeness of relationship in which all of these are one allows viewings from a different perspectives rather than clear separation.

The topical "divisions" approach women's lives and health from the perspective of the whole person across the lifespan. The approach is not only helpful and heuristic, but it is also corrective of former philosophical views of women as "other," as derivative or as deviant with respect to descriptions of personhood. These considerations are addressed, either directly or by implication, in those books entered in "Descriptions of Women." The section weaves together strands of religio-philosophical understandings, psychological concomitants, and medical ones. This approach is necessary and helpful since until quite recently women's health care has been provided in systems built upon understandings of the male person and the male body as normative. This approach has tended to result in perceiving gynecology as synonymous with women's health.

Concern for women's whole health across the lifespan is addressed under the topic "Care of Women," which considers current issues pertinent to women's health. This section annotates books which do not confuse women's health care with gynecology only. Neither do they tend to medicalize women's natural processes. In this chapter, one finds not only issues that have been clearly seen as medical, but also issues, both societal and work related, that are primary concerns, even in the health care professions, for women's whole health. The debate over whether there ought to be a women's health specialization, distinct from whole health for human persons, gender non-specific, is considered both on an overall level and as part of specific health issues such as cardiac concerns, osteoporosis, and breast cancer. This section attends to an overall movement of thirty years through shifts of emphases and across continents. Since women's health has become more clearly recognized as a global concern, the section includes recent publications concerning the Fourth United Nations Conference on Women held in Beijing in 1995.

Given more recent epistemological understandings and the progress of women in rediscovering their own history, both through recapturing what had not been included in history books and through researching more fully those inclusions which had been glossed over, it is important to spend time considering women's contributions in the healing professions. The topic "Care by Women," while it considers women's contributions in the Health Care Professions, makes the historical and sociological connections in terms of cultural and philosophical descriptions of women and current women's health concerns, by rejoining the caregiver and the cared for. Women have not been able to neatly separate these two, nor has society in general, for good or ill. This chapter includes books considering the family, most specifically, women as health care providers in that system, a concept and reality which needs to be remembered during the current crisis calling for health care reform. Among the contributions provided by women currently caring for the wellbeing of the healing professions are new curricula for medical schools. These will be considered as they also attempt a more integrated set of concerns.

"Self-Education and Self-Help" provides a sweeping approach to the women's health care movement over the past thirty years in the United States and Canada and moves the questions one more step, that is, to the issue of advocacy. The section pays attention to the demand for women's self-education in health care, tracing that movement from the first printing of *Our Bodies, Ourselves* by the Boston Women's Health Care Collective to its most recent publication.

The set of annotations supplied under "Costs and Benefits" entertains questions beyond the money issues in women and health to the literal economic issues, that is, those having to do with the Greek, *oeconomia,* management of a household, including the household of the state, and its Latin concomitant *vicus,* neighborhood. Thus, books are chosen which consider the larger issues of resource management and elucidate the larger payments society makes for nonattention to women and health, as well as the more proactive and positive benefits of whole person wellness for women.

Last, there is a full set of annotations on "Addictions," a concern which has been timely and relevant for at least the past twenty years. As the questions move from recovery per se to total wellness and past that to some more recent legal questions concerning women and pregnancy, it becomes appropriate to point toward useful information relevant for framing the pertinent questions.

Each topical division of this book is preceded by a brief introduction contextualizing the specific annotations. Some annotations will identify other books which might afford the reader particular benefit or enjoyment in being read in tandem with a specific entry. These "companion" books will be chosen only from entries elsewhere in this annotated bibliography. Author, title, publishing house and date will be included in the recommendation. Each of the approximately 300 full book entries, including some specific chapter annotations, is pertinent in some way to each of the other topics and to the integrated whole. No section is totally independent of the others, although each can be read and enjoyed for itself alone. Due to the interweaving of concerns for women's whole health, and given new epistemologies which have been largely driven by women's experience and research, a number of books will fit well in several categories. Having placed a given book in one of those several categories, I will attempt to make the reader aware of its multifaceted character. Where I have deemed it helpful, I have annotated specific chapters or essays in these books and placed them in chapters other than the one in which the full book appears.

While the entries are more heavily concentrated on works published in the United States and Canada, the entries do include international considerations. The individual voices in this choir of books sing in their own range even as they blend as one chorus. At any given point there is a beauty to be gained by hearing the individual air or counterpoint as well as by listening to the full harmony.

DESCRIPTIONS OF WOMEN

INTRODUCTION

The topic of women and health, cannot be addressed in a helpful manner without employing an interdisciplinary context. This chapter, focusing on descriptions of "woman" from that context, seeks to situate those descriptions in historical understandings, in religious and philosophical understandings, in psychological understandings, and in medical understandings. These understandings impinge one upon the other so that, at times, it becomes difficult to distinguish them one from the other. In those times when the distinction seems more clear, the interrelationship is such that the reader cannot understand the one without its concomitant meaning in the other. Thus, this set of annotations blends together books which either state directly descriptive definitions of women, or limn by implication such descriptions. It contains studies and insights published from the 1970s through the mid 1990s, scholarly works as well as popular ones.

Studies begun before the 1970s started to pay attention to women's historical contributions, sometimes by reading the silences and reconstructing women's contributions, sometimes by tracing documentary evidence and bringing it forth into the light. In both instances there was movement from the reality that women were being hidden from history to an awareness of women being hidden in history and thence to women being brought clearly into history's light. This book chooses to begin with works of the 1970s because they were built upon and bring out more clearly to the reader the discovery/rediscovery of the history of women. Folded into these histories are the understandings of women current in various eras.

Long-standing religious and philosophical traditions which defined "woman" as the derivative and non-normative human being drove histories and in turn were driven by them. Thus, religious and philosophical understandings are presented, some direct, some indirect. The interweaving connections between and among religion, philosophy, and history still present themselves in culture even when the articulated historical, philosophical, and religious definitions have changed. Until the changed descriptions are actually lived out for a long enough period, they remain present in the assumptions, feelings, and behaviors of society. Thus, they continue to impinge upon daily customs, research expectations and policies, allocation of funds, and allocation of status. All of these descriptions and expectations have an impact not only upon what we decide is "health" but what we decide is "women's health."

The need for presenting psychological as well as medical understandings of women then becomes clear. Because of male normativity in historical, philosophical, and religious concepts, decisions about what is medically and psychologically "normal" for women have tended to describe health and illness for us in particular ways consistent with those concepts. Sometimes the result has been overtreatment for some medical situations generally connected with women; sometimes it has been undertreatment for medical situations which pertain to women but are generally associated with men.

I have chosen not to label the books entered in this topical division by the distinct classifications of history, religion, philosophy, psychology, or medicine but rather to intermingle them so that the reader may have the felt impression that they are so interconnected as to describe whole sets of attitudes with which we deal as we consider women and health. Begun in the 1960s, these descriptions of women grew in the 1970s, flourished in the 1980s, and came to new integration in the 1990s. While the preponderance of annotations in this chapter deal with books published in the last three decades of the twentieth century, there are a few printed prior to that time. These shed light, by their very publication dates, on the long-standing nature of the issues.

Once this set of annotations supplies the context within which the issues are raised, the questions, data, and concepts of the following topical sections can be helpfully entertained. Generally speaking, those books published during the 1970s and the early 1980s focus on differences and remediation of old concepts, explaining conceptual lacks and making the case for women to be considered as persons and as full moral agents. Those books published in the late 1980s and the 1990s take a more proactive direction in terms of building up more integrated approaches, fostering the growth and implications of new concepts, working as though the former remediations are "done," even though in society at large these remain a "not yet." While these approaches are not alienated from each other, they are two distinct "colors" in the rainbow arc of understandings of women which lead to changed assumptions and behaviors vis-à-vis women and health.

ANNOTATIONS

Andolsen, Barbara H., Christine E. Gudorf, and Mary D. Pellauer, eds. *Women's Consciousness, Women's Conscience: A Reader in Feminist Ethics.* San Francisco: Harper and Row, 1985.

This collection of essays focuses on the interconnections among social, cultural, and economic structures and dominant notions of ethical behavior. It makes the case for the possibility of women's experience in those structures to serve as a basis for a new kind of ethics. While contributors offer a wide range of considerations, most of the essays concentrate on religious experience, most particularly the experience of women in traditional religions. Topics such as women's unpaid labor, violence against women, feminism and peace, female friendship, anti-Semitism, African American spirituality, sexuality, and procreative choice lead to the final section's essays outlining and theorizing about the development of a feminist ethics. Particularly helpful is a feminist theological critique of Christian ethics. One beauty of this book is the number of better known feminist writers on religion and spirituality, among them Starhawk, June Jordan, Judith Plaskow, and Rosemary Reuther. This roster provides the reader an opportunity to read other pertinent books with greater recognition and familiarity.

Armstrong, Karen. *The Gospel According to Women: Christianity's Creation of the Sex War in the West.* Garden City, NY: Anchor Press/Doubleday, 1987.

Written by a former Anglican nun, this critical history of women in Christianity uses classical theological writings and draws from the lives of women. It is a history of Christianity's oppression of women, categorizing them either as sinful (Eve) or saintly (Mary). Armstrong makes the case that sex has been the main problem of women in the Western world, a problem fostered by Christianity. Thus, she raises Christian approaches to that problem from within the myths, images, and history of that tradition. Armstrong provides a balance by raising both the damaging aspects of Catholicism and Protestantism as well as their positive aspects, drawing women to activism in social concerns. In looking at women in Christianity, both from the point of view of men's ways of regarding them and from the point of view of women's efforts to live within the framework of Christianity, Armstrong presents a tone and color readable to those within and outside the Christian traditions.

Backhouse, Constance, and David Flaherty, eds. *Challenging Times: The Women's Movement in Canada and the United States.* Montreal: McGill-Queen's University Press, 1992.

Arising from a joint project of the Center for Women's Studies and Feminist Research and the Center for American Studies, this book is a wonderfully interdisciplinary collection of essays combining history, theory, practical issues, and political concerns. It is quite helpful in that it covers both Canadian and United States perspectives, history, and concerns. The roster of its contributors is indicative of the diversity, both cultural and professional, that does justice to such an enterprise. A good deal of the history covered is in the lived experience of the book's contributors, adding quite an alive element for the reader. The table of contents itself evinces, by representation, the large concerns of the book, including as it does such topics as "The Interrelationship of Academic and Activist Feminism," "Racism and the Women's Movement," and "Women and the Economy."

Belenky, Mary F., Blyth M. Clinchy, Nancy R. Goldberger, and Jill M. Tarule. *Women's Ways of Knowing: The Development of Self, Voice, and Mind.* New York: Basic Books, 1986.

This study not only attempts to explain why women are at odds with traditional (read male) ways of knowing but also provides an epistemological breakthrough toward more integrated ways of knowing. By pointing out that our culture's dependence on notions of objectivity as the source of knowledge leaves women silent and voiceless, and by using interviews and questionnaires, the authors look for women's experience of voice. Basing their interpretation on theories like Carol Gilligan's idea of a "different voice," they emphasize their interviewees' use of subjective knowledge with the aim of developing a system of education that will further women's "connected knowing" and teaching. Describing the ways of knowing as "subjective knowledge," "procedural knowledge," and "constructed knowledge," the authors present discussions on "Family Life and the Politics of Talk," "Toward an Education for Women," and "Connected Teaching." Of particular interest are Appendix A, "Interview Schedule," and Appendix B, "Educational Dialectics."

Boulding, Elise. *The Underside of History.* Boulder, CO: Westview Press, 1976.

The beauty of this book lies not only in its historical data and treatment but also in its copyright date. Long before the current framing of the question of women's health from a medical systems perspective and before the current framing of women's whole health issues, Boulding placed a historical "Alternative Development Story" before the readers' eyes. In devoting the whole of her second chapter to "Dominance, Dimorphism, and Sex Roles" she frames the interpretive historical question so that the alternative story is no longer hidden from history. Instead, she uncovers what is hidden in history. Her descriptions of convent infirmarians, herbalists, and family medical practitioners reveal women's presence in the healing professions long before moderns or contemporaries recognized it. The revised edition of this book (Sage Publications, 1992) is a two-volume work.

Boxer, Marilyn J., and Jean H. Quataert, eds. *Connecting Spheres: Women in the Western World, 1500 to the Present.* New York: Oxford University Press, 1987.
Clustered in three historical eras: 1500-1750, 1750-1890, and 1890-1987 this collection of scholarly essays addresses a range of topics. The essays pertinent to each era are preceded by an editor's overview of the period, are each introduced by an abstract, and each offer suggestions for further reading. The manner in which the topics are approached provides an integrated sense of varying understandings of women through consideration of such issues as religion, science, marriage, and economy. Illustrations, figures, and tables add to the understandings presented.

Bridenthal, Renate, and Claudia Koontz, eds. *Becoming Visible: Women in European History.* Boston: Houghton Mifflin, 1977. Revised edition, 1987.
In this influential collection of essays, analyses of early egalitarian societies, of the classical and medieval periods, of witchcraft, of preindustrial capitalism, and of women's roles in the Russian revolution and in Nazi Germany provide a wide range of considerations. While the book uses the terminology of commonly recognized historical periods, Joan Kelly-Gadol's essay "Did Women Have a Renaissance?" makes the case that traditional ideas of historical periods often do not relate to women's experience. It is also helpful for the reader to notice the differences between the original and revised edition. Changes in the second reveal not only the authors' continuing thought but also changes in society in the intervening years.

Broverman, Inge K., Donald M. Broverman, et al. "Sex Role Stereotypes and Clinical Judgments of Mental Health." *Journal of Counseling and Clinical Psychology*, 34 (1970):1-7.

This study is important because it showed, in its time, the stereotypical descriptors used by professionals in the psychotherapeutic fields. Three groups of professionals, equally mixed in terms of gender, level of education, and therapeutic expertise, were asked to supply descriptors for (1) the healthy adult male, (2) the healthy adult female, and (3) the healthy adult, gender non-specific. By and large, the descriptors for healthy adult male and for healthy adult were congruent. The descriptors for healthy adult female were clearly not only different but also less desirable traits. The traits were also those ascribed to women and men in Western theological tradition and culture. One might conclude from the results that women's choice, in terms of being psychologically healthy, was to have female traits and not be a healthy adult, or to have healthy adult traits and to be a "male," a double bind since both were in some way either undesirable or punishable.

Brownmiller, Susan. *Femininity.* New York: Fawcett Columbine, 1985.
Attempting to do some hard reckoning with the concept of femininity, Brownmiller traces experiences, from infancy through girlhood into ongoing adulthood, of expectations expressed through such things as gifts, clothing, education, and fairy tales. These elements she shows to shore up the code called femininity, which she sees as a tradition of imposed limitations. According to Brownmiller, femininity demands more than biological femaleness and is upheld by continuing demonstrations of difference. Failure at demonstrating difference can be confused with lack of caring about men. Tracing femininity as a powerful aesthetic erected on a recogniton of powerlessness, Brownmiller shows its result in female against female competition. She organizes her chapters along practical and easily recognizable lines such as body, hair, voice, and clothes, and she "attempts rational analysis free of mystification" with regard to her topic.

Bullough, Vern L., Brenda Shelton, and Sarah Slavin. *The Subordinated Sex: A History of Attitudes Toward Women.* Athens: University of Georgia Press, 1988.

Starting with the basis of Western attitudes in ancient cultures and ending with the United States of the 1980s, this book follows a thread of the history of ideas concerning women. While it includes considerations on women and Christianity, it also supplies cross cultural history. In terms not only of history, but also of analysis and pointers in the direction of strategy, this book provides a broad spectrum. Particularly interesting to those from Western cultures is the chapter "Sex Is Not Enough: Women in Islam," which presents Islam as encouraging positive attitudes toward sexuality and eroticism; in the author's words, "sex-positive." In its history of Islam, through drawing on Muslim literature myths and traditions, the authors show that positive attitudes about sexuality do not necessarily mean positive attitudes toward women.

Canadian Research Institute for the Advancement of Women. *Canadian Women's Studies/Feminist Research* (Canada Studies Resource Guides, Second Series). Government of Canada: Minister of Supply and Services, 1993.
A short annotated bibliography of Canadian works in various areas of women's studies, printed in both English and French. The introduction points out that feminist research in Canada is challenging power relationships and structural inequalities as they intersect with the debates on nationalism and racism as well as the ways Canadian society constructs and deconstructs inclusion and exclusion. The book notes that such research not only is Canadian and international but also is intended to aid understanding so that people may act to change society. For those who may wonder what is the difference between feminist and conventional research, the introduction provides a useful list of some of the important elements in feminist research practice. The entries touch many topics in contemporary Canadian society, from both historical and current perspectives, and provide a basic list for those interested in the contributions women have made and continue to make to Canada's story.

Caputi, Jane. *Gossips, Gorgons & Crones: The Fates of the Earth*. Santa
Fe, NM: Bear & Company, 1993.

With a foreword by Paula Gunn Allen, this analysis of nuclear-age
culture provides a look at Native American, pre-patriarchal, and
feminist philosophies and encourages a return of female powers. Pointing
out the power of poetry and myth, Caputi advises conscious mythmaking
in order to willfully imagine possibilities other than those brought by
patriarchal nuclear myth, namely ones through a perspective that admits
and respects female powers. Her creative use of imagery from
contemporary culture points out the connections between nuclear
theology and practical/behavioral outcomes. Both her incisive word
studies and her recommendations in the images of gossip, gorgon, and
crone reveal present assumptive definitions of women and herald
old/new ones which create a window of hope into a new world.

Cooey, Paula M. *Religious Imagination and the Body: A Feminist
Analysis*. Oxford, England: Oxford University Press, 1994.

As a work of philosophical theology, this book is, according to the
author's stated intention, "critical, constructive and theoretical rather
than doctrinal." Thus, Cooey takes human reason as her chief
accountability yardstick. This approach is in distinction from taking
biblical or doctrinal authority as her criterion. In challenging
dualism, Cooey approaches each of the issues she raises in terms of the
relation between the religious imagination and the body. While this
may not necessarily mean the gendered female body, for the most part
Cooey takes that as her special concern. Chapter 6, "Mapping Religion,"
not only provides the conclusion for this book but also can well be
considered its context. The sections of the chapter attend to clear
descriptions of key concepts as well as insightful conclusions about their
interrelationship. All of these provide a new and enlightening focus for
understanding Cooey's subject. This book is well read in tandem with
The Cry of Tamar by Pamela Cooper-White (Fortress Press, 1995), and

Christianity, Patriarchy and Abuse, edited by Joanne Carlson Brown and Carole R. Bohm (The Pilgrim Press, 1990).

Countryman, L. William. *Dirt, Greed and Sex: Sexual Ethics in the New Testament and Their Implications for Today.* Philadelphia: Fortress Press, 1990.

Beginning with a consideration of Purity laws in the Judaeo-Christian scriptures, Countryman proceeds to a discussion of women and children as property and ends with a consideration of New Testament sexual ethics and a contemporary world: thus, his Part 1, "Dirt," Part 2, "Greed," and Part 3, "Sex." This book is particularly helpful in that the person who is not a professional scripture scholar can read and enjoy it and see inappropriate questions for what they are, contemporary issues read backwards into frameworks which no longer exist. Because he can sift these questions and interpretations, Countryman allows his readers the opportunity to see where, in fact, scriptural sexual ethics may fit today. This book is appropriate to an annotated bibliography on women and health because poor interpretations of scriptural sexual ethics over centuries have contributed to belief systems which see women neither as possessed of their own bodies nor as normative as human bodies.

Daly, Mary. *The Church and the Second Sex.* New York: Harper and Row, 1975.

Originally published in 1968, this critique of sexism in the Roman Catholic Church makes the case for radical transformation of what Daly labels "life-destroying" elements in that establishment. She points up the church's complicity in maintaining the secondary status of women in Catholic countries. This edition contains the author's new post-Christian introduction which rejects Christianity and shows how Daly's ideas have changed over time. It also contains a chapter by chapter critique of the book itself. While *Gyn/Ecology*, mentioned below, seems most pertinent for inclusion in this annotated bibliography, choosing to read Daly's subsequent books will afford the reader a chance to see the further development of her thought.

Daly, Mary. *Gyn/Ecology: The Metaethics of Radical Feminism.* Boston: Beacon Press, 1978.

Building upon and a leap forward from her own *Beyond God the Father* (Beacon Press, 1973) and *The Church and the Second Sex* (Beacon Press, 1975), Daly calls for exorcising patriarchal attitudes, habits, modes of thought, and world-views characterized by a male-centered theology. She encourages women to claim once again a woman-centered existence by putting in bold relief, and in a creatively unique approach to word meanings, the outcomes of patriarchal understandings. This radical feminist philosophy recaptures goddess traditions and is unafraid to use terminology associated with wicca. Its particular helpfulness in terms of women and health is in its ability to make connections between philosophical terminology and concepts and specific medical outcomes. Her considerations around therapy and gynecological issues created an opening of meaning with which women could reframe their health questions. The updated edition of this book (Beacon Press, 1990) contains a new introduction that is both witty and ironic, dealing with the author's experiences in 1975, when she began her work on the original edition of *Gyn/Ecology*. Bonnie Mann's appendix to the 1990 edition deals with the effects of this book upon the numbers of women who have read it.

Dixon-Mueller, Ruth. *Population Policy and Women's Rights: Transforming Reproductive Choice.* Westport, CT: Praeger, 1993.

In this work, Dixon-Mueller calls for a gathering of feminist forces to recognize the global problem of population levels, to articulate feminist principles on which responsive policy can be based, to build alliances, and to work for women to have a full range of reproductive rights and health. Feminists have been caught between antibirth proponents, seeking to control population, and probirth proponents, primarily nationalist and fundamentalist forces. She finds both these groups seeking to arrogate control of women's bodies. The essays in this book present the issues from the perspective of a feminist demographer. At the same time, they call for a sea change in thinking and a call to listen to the diverse voices of women of the world. The book has four parts interweaving history of ideas; human rights, both social and economic; and women's rights, including reproductive freedom. Chapter 5, "Women's Rights and Reproductive Choice: Rethinking the Connections," is a model case in point.

Eisler, Riane. *The Chalice and the Blade: Our History, Our Future*. San Francisco: Harper and Row, 1987.

Searching for answers to very large questions, Eisler's book differs from prior studies in that it works to embrace the whole of history, that is, prehistory as well as recorded history, and to embrace the whole of humanity, both male and female. She raises two alternatives as human possibilities: the *dominator*, or ranking model, and the *partnership*, or linking model. Taking her title, *The Chalice and the Blade*, from a turning point in prehistory when direction changed from a partnership to a dominator model, Eisler finds the contemporary human community standing at a crossroads. She finds the root of our problem in social systems which idealize the power of the Blade, the equation of power with dominance and violence, in short, the power of war and death. She finds light and insight in the power of the Chalice, life generating and nurturing power, woman-inspired and life-affirming. She points not only toward a rediscovery but also toward a contemporarily appropriate return to the partnership model. She does this through historical and sociological research which encourages a breakthrough in evolution. Eisler makes an interesting observation when she points out that, historically, the opposite of patriarchy has not been matriarchy; rather, it has been equality.

Faludi, Susan. *Backlash: The Undeclared War Against American Women*. New York: Doubleday/Anchor Books, 1991.

Dealing with the voices expressing ideas that women are enslaved and unhappy precisely because of their liberation, and that the women's movement has proven to be women's enemy, Faludi offers a huge amount of data put together with insight pointing out that this is not the case. Presenting the myths involved in such claims, Faludi considers the backlash in popular culture, the origins of these reactions, and the effect of backlash upon women's minds, jobs, and bodies. She provides information questioning whether women have "made it" to equality, the presupposition which has elicited backlash, and whether they "have it all" and the work of equality is, in fact, accomplished. Faludi sees the 1980s as a decade of backlash, which, though not an organized movement, is no less destructive. Faludi estimates that this backlash against women's rights succeeds to the degree that it appears not to be political.

Farmer, David Albert, and Edwina Hunter, eds. *And Blessed Is She: Sermons by Women.* San Francisco: Harper and Row, 1990.

Presented in two parts, "Women Preachers of the Past" and "Contemporary Women Preachers," this book shows that women have, in fact, been preaching from American beginnings. This was done many times outside the mainstream, so that while few have had formal pulpits, certainly they still preached. The selections cover a wide variety of topics and of styles, presenting such past preachers as Mother Lucy Wright, a Shaker leader; Anna Howard Shaw, a medical doctor who was the first woman ordained by the Methodist Protestant church; Aimee Semple McPherson, an evangelist; and Georgia Elma Harkness, the first woman to hold a professorship at a theological seminary. It also pays attention to present preachers, who may, in fact, be more familiar to the reader. They include Elizabeth Achtemeier, Rita Nakashima Brock, LaTaunya M. Bynum, Margaret Ann Cowden, Joan Delaplane, and Toinette Eugene. The introductions to each section and the ending bibliography are particularly helpful, providing both historical perspectives and differences in style and sources used by the preachers represented. This book dealing with histories of cogent women preachers provides forceful descriptions by actually including texts of these women's sermons.

Fausto-Sterling, Ann. *Myths of Gender: Biological Theories About Women and Men.* New York: Harper Collins, 1992.
This revised edition with a new chapter on brain anatomy, sex differences, and homosexuality looks at biological and anatomical issues without lapsing into biological determinism. Fausto-Sterling's ability to do excellent science and point toward its implications in social belief enhances a welcome discussion opening questions which can be prematurely closed by contemporary cultural habits. In the chapter on "Hormones and Aggression" the author does a fine job of showing the social implications of the sexual politics of science. In her last chapter,"Sex and Science," Fausto-Sterling points out that, given the lack of substance behind some ideas about biologically based sex differences, scientists can use observations/interpretations to bolster or to undermine common social beliefs and prejudices. One of the best contributions of this book is its readability for those who are not professional scientists, biological or social.

Fisher, Elizabeth. *Woman's Creation: Sexual Evolution and the Shaping of Society.* Garden City, NY: Anchor Press/Doubleday, 1979.
This work is an overview of human history from its earliest beginnings to the twentieth century. Fisher takes a female point of view in examining the earlier archaeological discoveries made by males as they ascribed their own prejudices and interpretations to various artifacts. She illustrates how the language used to describe human activity effectively obscures or eliminates women and their contributions to society. She also proposes an explanation of the development of patriliny and its resultant patriarchal patterns of domination, war, and violence, which are now so ingrained. Works such as this enable people to take a critical look at how men have written "our" early story.

Fox-Genovese, Elizabeth. *Within the Plantation Household: Black and White Women of the Old South.* Chapel Hill: University of North Carolina Press, 1988.
In charting this history of the experiences of black slave women and

white slave-owning women in the United States' South prior to the Civil War, the author presents the case that slave-owning women had too large an investment in their privileges to support abolition. Thus, she considers that only black women were true abolitionists. The author holds that slavery as an institution made it impossible for black and white women to form bonds of sisterhood. Drawing on both published and unpublished writings, Fox-Genovese uses a personal and imaginative style to examine notions of women's rights, attitudes toward slavery, sexuality, and the Civil War. The author provides a long and helpful bibliography.

Gerber Fried, Marlene, ed. *Abortion to Reproductive Freedom: Transforming a Movement.* Boston: South End Press, 1990.
This book is an anthology of articles from activists and academics involved in the fight for reproductive rights in the United States. It offers a critique and history of the abortion rights struggle from the 1960s on and argues for a more inclusive movement for reproductive rights that recognizes more fully difference and diversity. Ultimately, this anthology argues for expanding the abortion rights movement to a multicultural feminist one. In its very arrangement, the book makes the case for a greater cooperation between academics and activists. It is well read in tandem with Linda Gordon's Women's Body, Women's Right, (Grossman, 1977).

Gilligan, Carol. *In a Different Voice: Psychological Theory and Women's Moral Development.* Cambridge, MA: Harvard University Press, 1982.
In this once controversial feminist analysis of women's psychology. Gilligan argues that women base moral decisions on an ethic of care, while men base them on abstract justice. Much of this book's importance lies in the response it originally aroused, with critics claiming that Gilligan's sample was too small and that her thesis rested on questionable assumptions. Others saw it as an important way of championing values traditionally held by women and of overcoming

Western culture's dehumanizing emphasis on competition and other "masculine" values. In fact, dealing with psychological theory and women's development ultimately does have implications for ethics. Gilligan's postulate that women view moral problems in terms of conflicting responsibilities to self and others eventuates in a reflective understanding of care as a central guide to resolving the conflict. Whatever the response has been, the book's contribution is validated in the ongoing talk centered around an ethic of care. The importance of *In a Different Voice* for this bibliography is in its opening the way for considerations of an "ethic of care" as appropriate to nursing, to ministry, and to medicine.

Gilman, Charlotte Perkins. *Women and Economics*. Boston: Small, Maynard & Co., 1898.

The author begins by noting that humans are the only animal species in which "an entire sex lives in a relation of economic dependence on the other "that the economic relation is combined with the sex relation" (p. 5). She continues that "while motherhood is the ground that prevents her from working, it is rather the hours she spends on extra-maternal unpaid duties which would suffice to provide her economic independence were she employed." Contemporary discussions concerning women and retirement issues might find this pertinent.

Gordon, Linda. *Women's Body, Women's Right: A Social History of Birth Control in America*. New York: Grossman, 1977.

This book was the first comprehensive history of birth control in the United States. Gordon identifies three major phases in the movement, each expressing the interests of a different group of women. During the late nineteenth century, activists in favor of "voluntary motherhood" called for abstinence or contraception to help women, thus freed from constant childbearing, to devote themselves to the raising of children. From 1910 to 1920 separate contraception oriented organizations were developed. During the 1940s and afterward, liberal reform centered around "planned parenthood," more akin to contemporary notions of birth control. In examining controversies over contraception, population control, and abortion, Gordon argues that reproductive freedom is central to women's freedom.

Graff, Ann O'Hara, ed. *In the Embrace of God: Feminist Approaches to Theological Anthropology.* Maryknoll, NY: Orbis Press, 1995.
This collection of theological essays pulls together, in a very readable manner, important insights and their applications from a decade's work of redefining what it is to be human from a theological standpoint. Multicultural in its approach and the variety of its essays, *In the Embrace of God* addresses such issues as the history of feminist theology, hearing women's voices, interpreting women's experience, constructing culturally based feminist theologies, coping with suffering, and reflecting upon ecofeminism. The essays show the challenges of feminist theology to reconstruct more authentic theological anthropologies while, at the same time, keeping alive the concrete and diverse experiences of women.

Graham, Elaine. *Making the Difference: Gender, Personhood and Theology.* Minneapolis, MN: Fortress Press, 1996.
Noting the changes in relationships between men and women in contemporary Western society, the author also shows that Western religious traditions have been affected by these. Spurred by these societal changes, religious groups have been required to reexamine their teachings and practices. A significant phenomenon in Western Christianity during the last generation has been the growth of feminism and of feminist theology. This book examines the debate over the meaning and the import of gender, of gender difference, and of the social construction of gender. In considering these categories, Graham lays out how gender is understood in the social sciences and draws out its pertinence for theology and for religion. In Part I, she considers "Gender Issues," in Part II, "Gender Disciplines," and in Part III, "Gender Themes." Particularly telling for the reader consulting this annotated bibliography are Chapter 9, "Knowledge: Feminist Epistemologies and

Philosophies of Science," and Chapter 10, "Making the Difference: Towards a Theology of Gender." This last chapter is particularly helpful in its offering of a new paradigm for integrating theories of gender into Christian theology and practice, a paradigm that limns an agenda for further studies.

Grahn, Judy. *Blood, Bread, and Roses: How Menstruation Created the World.* Boston: Beacon Press, 1993.
With a foreword by Charlene Spretnak this book provides an exploration of folklore, myth, religion, anthropology, and history and makes the case for male origin stories to be balanced by a recognition of women's central role in the shaping of civilization. Grahn does this as a poet theorizing with an associative mind, speculating that the foundation of many origin stories   is the "menstrual mind," the crossing from primate consciousness to the development of abstracting and conceptualizing consciousness. This development was based on women's awareness that the menstrual cycle is related to the rhythm of the moon. Grahn's discussion of "parallel menstruations" provides an insightful set of lenses which also give vision for constructing a new set of rites. This book provides a description of women different from what is usually expected in contemporary culture.

Gross, Rita M. *Feminism and Religion: An Introduction.* Boston: Beacon Press, 1996.
Spanning the feminist revolution of the past three decades, this book examines the changes not only in women's religious lives, but also in ideas about religion itself. Delving into the history of women in the major religions of the world, including prepatriarchal ones, the author looks at feminist transformations of theology, leadership, ritual, and institutions in Judaism, Islam, and Christianity as well as Buddhism, Hinduism, and feminist spirituality. She traces feminist investigations into these aspects and critiques several feminist visions of the future of religion. The book is not only balanced but also wide ranging in its considerations. In its raising to attention the accomplishments of feminist

approaches to the study of religion over a twenty-five year period, this book is encouraging as well as provocative.

Haddad, Yvonne Y., and Ellison B. Findly, eds. *Women, Religion and Social Change*. Albany: State University of New York Press, 1985.
These essays, on women and the formation of religious tradition, on social change and women's role in religious institutions, and on women, religion, and revolution, supply historical and contemporary cases in point. The book includes Christianity, Hinduism, Buddhism, Judaism, and Islam in its considerations. The introduction, by Nancy Falk, highlights structural parallels between religion and revolutionary movements, making the case for the Marxist class struggle to be another picture of the struggle between good and evil. The book has an interdisciplinary character, including essays on roles of women in the development of religions, images and symbols of women in religious art, and religious aspects of women's participation in the Nicaraguan revolution as well as the United States abolition movement.

Haddon, Genia Pauli. *Body Metaphors: Releasing God-Feminine in Us All*. New York: Crossroads, 1988.
Haddon proposes a different paradigm of masculinity and femininity and discredits stereotypical definitions by attempting to "reground" those understandings in the "authority of body differences." By the use of "God-feminine," the author, an ordained minister and psychotherapist, intends to emphasize the roots in masculinist God-religion of a newly emerging God image. She encourages an understanding of God as the One in whose image female identity is modeled, without reviving an ancient prepatriarchal deity. Grounding her conclusions in reflections on physiology which are far from the commonly understood stereotypes concerning male and female bodies, Haddon attempts a new integration. Her chapters 9, 10, and 11, "The Body That Bleeds but Is Not Wounded," "Gift of the Thirteenth God-Mother," and "Delivered by the Crone," offer reflectively insightful physiological considerations ending in an extremely positive approach to menopause and a hope of society's

honoring of the wisdom of the Crone. In opening reflections upon the feminine and masculine aspects in each human, Haddon suggests that women and men can encounter the Feminine Divine through meditation, therapy, and liturgy.

Heyward, Carter. *Staying Power: Reflections on Gender, Justice, and Compassion.* Cleveland, OH: The Pilgrim Press, 1995.

In her preface, "Re-Imagining Justice," Heyward sets the tone and context of her book, considering language, justice, and relation. She forms an *inclusio* with Chapter 14, "Re-Imagining: A Conversation - Carter Heyward and Beverly Harrison." This conversation between two ethicists enfleshes the passionately presented concepts in the first thirteen chapters, conversation being an apt metaphor for Heyward's message. Constantly intertwining the themes of gender, justice, and compassion, this Episcopal priest makes a contribution to the dismantling of heteropatriarchy by encouraging the reclaiming of body and of eros. Her continued call for experience, experiment, and quest of right relationship rings clear throughout her chapters. A beauty of the author's writing is that she anchors her concepts with clear and concrete experiences of people and life events which display her message. Heyward's endnotes contain explanations as well as citations, offering the reader a richness of understanding. Her bibliography affords excellent direction for further reading.

Heyward, Carter. *Touching Our Strength: The Erotic as the Power and the Love of God.* San Francisco: Harper and Row, 1989.

This theological enterprise encourages the renewal of the recognition of the sacred aspect of sexuality. Calling for a wholeness of relationships, it creates a theology of lesbian and gay relationships, calling for sexuality with honor rather than domination. Calling forth the relational matrix of being human, Heyward combines the historical, the ethical, and the religious, to describe sex and God as "empowering sparks of ourselves in relation" (p. 3). She attempts to provide voice for an embodied sense of relationship among persons experiencing their sexualities as liberating and justice-oriented resources. Linking patterns of sexual and gender injustice with other structures of relationship, such as race and economics, Heyward points toward a transformative mode of right relationship. Her final chapter, "Undying Erotic Friendship: Foundations for Sexual Ethics," contains a list of twelve healing commitments which demand reflective energy as well as concrete behavior change for United States society.

Hinsdale, Mary Ann, and Phyllis Kaminski, eds. *Women and Theology.* Annual Publication of the College Theology Society, Volume 40. Maryknoll, NY: Orbis Press, 1994.
This book is a collection of essays, focused through the lens of theology as conversation and clustered in three parts: "Entering the Conversation," "Adding Voices," and "Changing the Terms." The essays interweave experiential considerations as well as theoretical ones, individual expressions as well as multicultural context, a call for solidarity as well as culturally based theologies, church issues as well as world issues, and distinctly feminist concerns as well as a move for a new integration beyond gender. This fortieth anniversary volume of the annual publication of the College Theology Society includes, as afterword, the Presidential Address given by Joan A. Leonard, a quite readable piece contextualizing the focus of the fortieth convention of the society. The collection as a whole and each essay in particular are well read in tandem with *In The Embrace of God*, edited by Ann O'Hara Graff (Orbis Press, 1995).

Holmes, Helen B., and Laura M. Purdy, eds. *Feminist Perspectives in Medical Ethics.* Bloomington: Indiana University Press, 1992.
Opening this collection of essays with "A Call to Heal Medicine" and "A Call to Heal Ethics," the editors place the ensuing discussions in context. The collection is then divided into five groupings, "The Medical Ethics Community: Feminist Views," "The Role of Caring in Health Care," "Women and Clinical Experiments," "Women and New Reproductive 'Choices'," and "Contract Pregnancy." Each of the essays

views its concerns from the large perspectives of philosophy, science, and understandings of women. The essays deal with concrete issues, each of which is of specific concern to women's health, dignity, and well-being. Each essayist's gift for placing her question involves pertinent data, as well as insightful connections which put implications in bold relief and make them accessible, not only for those in the field but also for interested people who are neither ethicists nor medical professionals. This book is one helpful backdrop for reading any book specifically concerned with a given women's health issue.

Hubbard, Ruth. *The Politics of Women's Biology.* New Brunswick, NJ: Rutgers University Press, 1990.

In this exploration of the relationship between science and political decision making, Hubbard finds "women's biology" to be a social construct and a political concept rather than a scientific one. She mentions pertinent nineteenth century data with regard to women's attempts at access to higher education. The reader can enjoy this book alongside Susan Sherwin's No Longer Patient, (Temple University Press, 1992).

Hubbard, Ruth. *Profitable Promises.* Monroe, ME: Common Courage Press, 1995.

This book is in three parts: "The Link Between Genes, Illness and Behaviors," "Women, Science and Power," and "Toward a Political Understanding of Science." Most of the essays have been or are in the process of being published elsewhere. Some draw on previous work with Elijah Wald, *Exploding the Gene Myth* (Beacon Press, 1993). Part I builds on *The Politics of Women's Biology* (Rutgers University Press, 1990) and on *Exploding the Gene Myth.* Hubbard shows how the concept of the healthy or asymptomatic ill draws attention from major health issues which needlessly threaten huge segments of the human community. Part II illustrates ways in which often prestigious scientists, physicians, and legal experts use their expert knowledge to reinforce, or at least support, conservative opinions about women's place in society.

Part III shows that scientists are not detached, objective observers: Culture shapes interests and commitments. What gets omitted in public discourse is that scientists set the terms of the experiments. To do that they make choices affected by economic constraints, cultural biases, personal history, and position and role in culture.

Isasi-Diaz, Ada Maria. *En La Lucha: An Hispanic Women's Theology.* Minneapolis, MN: Fortress Press, 1993.
As she gathers Hispanic women's everyday religious experience and practice, gives them expression, discerns key themes, and returns them to the Hispanic and larger theological communities as sources of power, enablement, and enrichment, Isasi-Diaz displays a courage and cultural base. This work is a grounded contribution to women's theological diversity.

Johnson, Elizabeth A. *She Who Is: The Mystery of God in Feminist Theological Discourse.* New York: Crossroad, 1994.
In a lucid synthesis of feminist wisdom and classical theological sources, Johnson offers a strikingly coherent feminist theology able to invite and encourage a new and renewed vision of Christianity. This book is well read in dialogue with the work of Mary Daly, more particularly her later books. While there is some commonality of concerns and insights, the tonality and conclusions differ so as to provide the reader a set of options for help in deciding where s/he stands.

Johnson, Elizabeth A. *Women, Earth, and Creator Spirit.* New York: Paulist Press, 1993.
The 1993 Madeleva Lecture in Spirituality, this book explores the thesis that exploitation of the earth is connected to the marginalization of women and that both are connected to forgetting the Creator Spirit. Rethinking these three - women, earth, and Creator Spirit - Johnson proceeds by considering major issues. Chapter 1, "The Crisis: Ecocide," provides a look at the current ecological situation. Chapter 2, "A Taproot of the Crisis: The Two-Tiered Universe," examines the rationality of

hierarchical dualism. Chapter 3, "Hearkening to Women's Wisdom," Chapter 4, "Discerning Kinship with the Earth," and Chapter 5, "Remembering Creator Spirit," offer considerations on the neglected sources of wisdom which contain the possibilities for an alternative vision. Johnson's conclusionary chapter, "Conversion to the Circle of Earth," not only recalls the purpose and work of this book but also has a poetic and motivational tone which contextualizes her discussion.

Jordan, Judith V., Alexandra G. Kaplan, Jean Baker Miller, Irene P. Striver, and Janet L. Surrey. *Women's Growth in Connection: Writings from the Stone Center.* New York: The Guilford Press, 1991.
Divided into two parts, "A Developmental Perspective" and "Applications," this collection of essays provides an overarching description of women as relational beings whose organizing factor is relational growth. The authors have, as one of their central critiques of existing developmental theory, its bias toward independence, separation, autonomy, and self-sufficiency. Thus, in Part I, they present some of their beginning principles in portraying women. In Part II, they apply their formulations to specific topics such as work, eating disorders, and therapeutic implications of their relational model. The integrated quality of each essay makes it readable on its own as well as part of a larger whole. Woven throughout the essays is sufficient historical and theoretical consideration as to make this book understandable to a public beyond the professional therapeutic community.

Kaledin, Eugenia. "Mothers and More: American Women in the 1950s." In Barbara Haber, ed. *American Women in the Twentieth Century.* Boston: Twayne/G. K. Hall, 1984.
In this history of women's experience during a decade sometimes characterized in terms of suburban motherhood and its trapping of women, Kaledin argues that women in the 1950s were not merely victims but many times genuinely satisfied because they cherished a sense of "separate but equal" spheres. She also emphasizes women's career achievements in the arts, describing many of the decade's

successful women as "gifted outsiders." Chapters address education, work, women and politics, women writers and artists, African American women, and health issues. The book also provides helpful illustrations and figures.

Kessler-Harris, Alice. *Out to Work*. New York: Oxford University Press, 1982.
This book, a history of wage-earning women in the United States, explores the transformation of women's work into wage labor in the United States. Kessler-Harris attempts to illuminate the relationship between wage-earning and family roles, their tensions as well as their mutually reinforcing aspects. She considers how the waged work of women simultaneously sustained the patriarchal family and set in motion the tensions that are breaking it down. This book provides a new look at labor force patterns from the perspectives of women and sex role definitions, from colonial economy to the radical consequences of incremental change. Kessler-Harris' work is a good historical backdrop to the current state of the question of women and waged work, since women's workloads and economic status together provide the largest women's health care issues internationally, that is, overwork, underpay, and low ascribed status.

Kramarae, Chris, and Dale Spender, eds. *The Knowledge Explosion: Generations of Feminist Scholarship*. New York: Teachers' College Press, 1992.
A testimony to the scholarship and achievements of Women's Studies over the last decades, this book is a collection of multidisciplinary essays, with an introduction setting its framework It is a celebration as well as a stocktaking enterprise. Each essay deals with the place of women in its discipline twenty years ago, identifying feminist protests and critiques of the discipline, seeking to name the basic tenets of the discipline which have denied the experience of or discriminated against women, pointing out the new research priorities or directions emerging from feminist activity, discussing changes in the discipline, assessing the

contribution of feminist knowledge to the discipline, and assessing the current situation. The result is quite a readable book with something for each reader and an interconnectedness that helps to establish a sense of ease with the enterprise.

Larrington, Carolyne, ed. *The Feminist Companion to Mythology.* London: Pandora Press, 1992.
Holding that myth furnishes a new way to look at social structures, Larrington uses myths to examine constants and variables in the organization of human society. Myth, having conditioned the way we think about ourselves, has been appropriated by politicians as well as artists to tell us where we are and where we have come from. Larrington thus uses this study of myth to examine women's roles across cultures and historical periods. Keeping her definition of myth flexible, the author allows for legend and folk tale. She divides her book, a collection of essays, into six parts, honoring different times and cultures: Part 1, "The Near East," Part 2, "European," Part 3, "Asia," Part 4, "Oceania," Part 5, "America," and Part 6, "Goddesses in the Twentieth Century." The span of this book and the readability of its essays is particularly helpful It can be well read in dialogue with several of the essays in Charlene Spretnak's *Politics of Women's Spirituality* (Anchor Press/Doubleday, 1982).

Leavitt, Judith W. *Brought to Bed: Childbearing in America, 1750-1950.* New York: Oxford University Press, 1986.
Supporting her arguments through a broad range of firsthand accounts from women, including those taken from eighteenth and nineteenth century documents, Leavitt deals with the historical significance of childbirth. Two hundred years previous to 1950, childbirth in the United States was dangerous but women were in charge of its setting. By 1950, while childbirth had become less dangerous, women had surrendered control of the experience to physicians. Leavitt argues that in choosing to allow physicians to become the managers of childbirth, hardly did women anticipate what little power they would retain. In

dealing with her topic, Leavitt restores historical agency to women and gives a sympathetic account of physicians' difficulties. She addresses change in medical practice, the ideological aspect of science, and the place of childbearing in women's lives. Her book ends with 1950, on the edge of another change in birthing history, that of the natural childbirth movement.

Lerner, Gerda. *The Creation of Feminist Consciousness: From the Middle Ages to Eighteen-Seventy*. New York: Oxford University Press, 1993.
This is the second volume of Gerder Lerner's *Women and History* project. Her work in the first volume, *The Creation of Patriarchy*, dealt with that creation as taking place prior to the formation of Western civilization. Showing how the metaphors of gender constructed the male as the norm and the female as the deviant, she had shown that women had a relationship to the historical process different from that of men. In this volume, Lerner focuses on certain basic themes. Having noticed that religion was the primary arena within which women fought for hundreds of years for feminist consciousness, Lerner includes the chapter "One Thousand Years of Feminist Biblical Criticism" in her set of chapters beginning with "The Educational Disadvantaging of Women" and ending with "The Search for Women's History." In her conclusion, having seen women as "thinkers and creators of ideas," she posits that women can "reclaim the freedom of our minds as we reclaim our pasts."

Lerner, Gerda. *The Creation of Patriarchy*. New York: Oxford University Press, 1986.
Concerned that much of the work of modern feminism had been ahistorical, Lerner, as a women's history specialist, undertook her work. Seeing women's history as indispensable to their emancipation, she set about dealing with the conflict-ridden and highly problematic relationship of women to history. In returning the past of half, and sometimes more than half, of the human community to its own history, Lerner created a large historical framework within which women could

percieve and take ownership of that history. While women had always been central to the process of history, that is, had made history, they had been kept not only from knowing that history but also from the process of making meaning of it, that is, its ordering and interpretation. Lerner's arguments concerning the historicity of female subordination was an important step in the creation of new modes of analysis.

Lowe, Marian, and Ruth Hubbard, eds. *Women's Nature: Rationalizations of Inequality*. New York: Pergamon Press, 1983.
This book, examining what the authors consider false descriptions of women's nature and the concomitant limits to women's participation in society, looks toward an opening up of constrained self-views and outer visions for a better future. These myths about women's nature become more obvious as one sees the inconsistencies between these descriptions used to oppress women and the reality of the lives of individual women and groups of women. The chapter by Marian Lowe, on "Biology and Culture," and the one by Elizabeth Fee, "Women's Nature and Scientific Objectivity," situate these descriptors and their implications in the world of science. Of particular help in this collection are those essays which pertain to Black and to Indian women. These were published at a time when some were still accusing feminist concerns as being only those of white middle-class women.

McFague, Sallie. *The Body of God: An Ecological Theology*. Minneapolis, MN: Fortress Press, 1993.
In this work, McFague's organic model for conceiving God joins body with soul and humans with nature. It is a corrective to spiritualized, body-hating theologies, which have, by and large, been misogynist ones. Over a period of years, women friendly theologies have led to ecological ones. In her previous book, *Models of God* (Fortress Press, 1987), McFague had presented the models of God, mother, lover, and friend of the world. This focus on embodiment eventuated, in a way, in another model, her organic one which encourages the reader "to think and act as if bodies matter." While the author does not directly analyze body

oppressions, such as sexual discriminationand physical or sexual abuse, her model is a complement to these analyses. Chapter 2, "The Organic Model," critiques organic models in the classical form, models which have been hierarchical, anthropocentric, and androcentric. Her version from the sciences and from feminism suggests different possibilities. She stresses radical interrelationship and interdependence of all bodies even as she underscores their radical differences.

McKenny, Gerald P., and Jonathan R. Sande, eds. *Theological Analyses and the Clinical Encounter.* Boston: Kluwer Academic Publishers, 1994.

The introduction to this book considers theology, ethics, and the clinical encounter. Presented in three sections "The Medical Covenant Past, Present, and Future," "Principles in Revision," and "Beyond Principles" the work devotes four pages directly to women's health. Those considerations are housed in the essay "Empowerment in the Clinical Setting" by Karen Lebacqz. The size and placement of this discussion is a fine metaphor for what is still the state of affairs in mainline medical ethics and mainline theological pursuit. In her essay, Lebacqz considers that as one may learn justice from considering experiences of injustice, so one may discover something about empowerment by considering disempowerment. She mentions the 1991 film *The Doctor* as an instance of a male physician and surgeon experiencing disempowerment in the hospital setting. She includes the non-focus upon and non-treatment of women's issues as another subtle form of disempowerment, as well as problems of access to the clinical setting. Lebacqz calls for alternative structures so that empowerment can mean not only self-advocacy and participation in decisions significant to the patient but also receiving care from a system which is radically reoriented.

Matthews, Glenna. *The Rise of the Public Woman: Woman's Power and Woman's Place in the United States, 1630-1970.* New York: Oxford University Press, 1992.

Pointing out that public man and public woman have two different connotations in Western culture, Matthews, a historian, derives her insights by looking at history from an unusual angle. Noting that even by the end of the nineteenth century women had rather a tenuous claim on the public space, she shows a link between public female visibility and sexuality, that is, a separation of women into respectable and not respectable, with publicly visible meaning not respectable. She finds that while the work of a number of pioneers opened up the public space to women, there is, as yet, no real symmetry between the understanding of public man and that of public woman. In stating this reality, Matthews cites examples from the perspectives of race, class, religion, and ethnicity. Her division of public into legal, political,cultural, and spatial, or social geographic, is not only helpful but also clarified by her use of concrete instances which mirror the elements of this division. The author raises the question of relationship between the home and the world, noting that there is a lack of practical ways of melding justice for women with provision for the private sphere. She also sees a lack of political theory affording anything more than superficial attention to fostering private life.

Melosh, Barbara, ed. *Gender and American History Since 1890*. London: Routledge, 1993.
A collection of essays, this work illustrates early modern life and attitudes toward women in the United States. Already, at the turn of the twentieth century, as more and more young women remained single and worked, their wages were insufficient to live independently. The essays look at attitudes toward women in succeeding decades through the windows of art, literature and the developing consumer culture. Those essays considering the 1940s discuss the ways women assumed and then had to give up the freedom afforded them during   World War II by being immediately removed from segments of the paid labor force when the war was over. Racism is also dealt with in an essay considering Ida B. Wells' efforts to challenge white middle-class concepts and descriptions of "real" men and women.

Miller, Jean Baker. *Toward a New Psychology of Women.* Boston: Beacon Press, 1976.

This early and influential examination of female psychology stresses women's subordinate social position. In it, Miller argues that conflicts between unequals leads members of the subordinate group to develop indirect ways of behaving. As she describes the impact of subordination on thought processes and ways of conceptualizing, Miller emphasizes the importance of women beginning with their own experience rather than with rules of subordination. She encourages accepting conflict as a basic (read growth-producing) process. Miller's work was an early impetus to major breakthroughs in women's psychology. The revised edition of this book (1986) has a new foreword and epilogue. Chapter 11, "Reclaiming Conflict," adds a section on "Conflict Among Women Today."

Morawski, Jill G. *Practicing Feminisms, Reconstructing Psychology: Notes on a Liminal Science.* Ann Arbor: The University of Michigan Press, 1994.

This book, which the author describes as an "extended, multifocal essay," takes the positive stance of limning out new and evolving contours of feminist psychology. Choosing to be involved in making a new and different science, rather than to take a defensive or even corrective stance vis-à-vis the old scientific order, Morawski deals with objectivity, subjectivity, and validity in new and promising ways. She does this through an accomplished cultural analysis from within both feminism and psychology. In taking this contextualized stance, Morawski employs social epistemology as a new foundation for inquiry. She thus creates a situation where feminist psychology can be seen and apppreciated as a transformative science using reflexivity in cultural analysis to arrive at new psychological knowledge. Her first two chapters, "Feminism and Psychologies" and "Betwixt and Between," set a helpful context for reading the following chapters.

Numbers, Ronald L., and Darrel W. Amundsen, eds. *Health and Medicine in the Western Religious Traditions.* New York: Macmillan, 1986.

This book is a collection of primarily historical essays, showing connections between religion and medicine. It admits that many health-seeking individuals will tend to draw upon a spate of options made available to them in a spiritual heritage. While the book makes no distinction betweeen spirituality and religion, in practicality conflating these, it offers a rich set of considerations. It seeks to explore guiding visions and values embodied in faith traditions. It does, indirectly, offer descriptions of women by having some things to say about some of their roles in the history of healing in several Western traditions. This book, the first of two, is the companion to *Healing and Restoring*, edited by Laurence E. Sullivan (Macmillan, 1989).

Plant, Judith, ed. *Healing the Wounds: The Promise of Ecofeminism.* Toronto: Between the Lines, 1989.
A collection of articles, interviews, and poems, this work points out the connections between the oppression of women and the exploitation of the environment. It considers feminist activism in favor of the environment on an international level, highlighting the spiritual basis of ecofeminism and positing the presence of the goddess in nature. The contributors are from diverse backgrounds and include Ursula LeGuin, Starhawk, and Vandana Shiva.

Plaskow, Judith. *Sex, Sin and Grace.* New York: University Press of America, 1980.
The subtitle, *Women's Experience and the Theologies of Reinhold Niebuhr and Paul Tillich*, betrays the meaning of this first feminist dissertation out of Yale Divinity School. In this volume, Plaskow makes the case for what others in theology and across disciplines would point out, that the theological enterprise was predicated upon the experience of men. Her treatment of sin and human selfhood points up the fact that selfhood was defined in terms of men's self and its concomitant representation of sin as self-assertion, self-centeredness, and pride, likely sins for men. The temptations of women qua women could not be encompassed by "pride" and "will to power" but rather more likely by

triviality, distractability, and diffuseness. In other words, Plaskow found Niebuhr and Tillich guilty of identifying their important, but limited, male perspective with universal truth. There has been much water under the bridge since Plaskow's treatment, but it is a timely (not yet finished) and historical consideration opening the way for many questions to follow, questions upon which rest current notions of women's whole health in the face of the still not totally changed normativity of maleness = humanness in theology, pastoral care, medicine, and health care.

Raymond, Janice. *A Passion for Friends: Toward a Philosophy of Female Affection.* Boston: Beacon Press, 1986.
This is a feminist history and analysis of female friendship, including but not limited to lesbian relationships. Raymond emphasizes women's networks, including nuns and Chinese marriage resisters, as a means of resisting male domination. She outlines traditional obstacles to female friendships, among them popular assumptions about women's rivalry and the idea that women's most important relationships are necessarily those with men. Showing that a vision of female friendship with men is also necessary and central to achieving women's freedom, Raymond presents a large and encompassing picture. Woven throughout her insights are descriptions of women which have been held as well as descriptions of women which could be.

Rosser, Sue. *Women's Health—Missing from U.S. Medicine.* Bloomington: Indiana University Press, 1994.
Exploring the critiques resulting from male-focused medical research and health care practice and those solutions available to medical education which move women to share in the central focus, Rosser raises the importance of descriptions of women through Part One, "Critiques of the Androcentric Focus in Clinical Research and Practice." She concretely addresses women's differences in Part Two, "Ignoring Diversity Among Women in Clinical Research and Practice," and offers solutions in Part Three, "Including Women in Medical Education." This book synthesizes the historical, the ethical, and the medical while taking

a proactive and projective stance. It pays attention to newer epistemologies within which to understand the past and to reframe future possibilities. Particularly helpful is Chapter 2, "Underdiagnosis and Inadequate Treatment: AIDS and Women," as a specific case in point for viewing the results of androcentric bias in clinical research and practice.

Rothman, Barbara. *The Tentative Pregnancy: Prenatal Diagnosis and the Future of Motherhood*. London: Pandora Press, 1988.
This United States study not only explores the experiences of women undergoing prenatal testing but also provides a unique account of the impact of these new technologies on women's reproductive awarenesses. In the process of exploration the authors highlight ethical and social dilemmas that are often ignored by doctors and policy makers. In discussing the social and ethical implications of prenatal diagnosis, Rothman points out the difficulty for women in refusing the test when doctors and others urge it, arguing that prenatal diagnosis changes the experience of pregnancy. She calls this "difficult social state" in which women find themselves until about the twentieth week the "tentative pregnancy."

Sherwin, Susan. *No Longer Patient*. Philadelphia: Temple University Press, 1992.
In this feminist approach to bioethics the author shows that a feminist ethics of health care must ask its questions regarding health care practices with attention to the overall power structures of dominance and subordination. Chapter 9, "Ascriptions of Illness," considers how the construction of a medicalized view of women's experience assumes proprietorship over women's lives, while Chapter 10, "Medical Constructions of Sexuality," shows how medicine can play a key role in control of women. In tandem, these chapters limn clearly the power and implications of descriptions of women. The book itself reveals an integrative approach in its tripartite construction: Part One; "Theoretical Beginnings" Part Two; "Traditional Problems in Health Care Ethics" Part Three; "Feminist Expansions of the Bioethics Landscape."

Spelman, Elizabeth V. *Inessential Woman: Problems of Exclusion in Feminist Thought.* Boston: Beacon Press, 1988.

A look at the view of women in the writings of Plato, Aristotle, *The Second Sex* of Simone de Beauvior, and the work of Nancy Chodorow, this book shows how, in their critiques, feminists have developed a view of women that is white, middle-class, and American. Thus, any other woman is less than essential. Spelman discusses gender, race, class, and culture as she examines the writers' works and suggests that these aspects cannot be ignored if the resulting blindness supports male or white experience and culture. Spelman encourages the development of imagination and the gaining of knowledge, and then, the use of imagination to expand one's consciousness and tolerance, so that women's voices will be heard, for "though all women are women, no woman is only a woman" (p. 1).

Spretnak, Charlene, ed. *The Politics of Women's Spirituality: Essays on the Rise of Power Within the Feminist Movement.* Garden City, NY: Anchor Press/Doubleday, 1982.

This collection of essays treats pre-patriarchal and post-patriarchal, women-centered spirituality. This approach is proactive in that it does not devote energy to critiquing traditional religious denominations but rather offers experiences, thoughts, and insights revealing women's personal power. In naming connections between spirituality and politics the essays combine theoretical with practical tones. The collection deals with descriptions of women, by having the essayists name their own descriptions and nature through their writing. The overall introduction gives a good sense of the scope of women's spirituality, while the introductions to each part of the book set the context for each of the series of essays. The parts of the book move from past to future, from discovery to transformation. While the essays focus from varying perspectives (art, mythology, history, ethics) and are thematically bound together, each essay can also be read on its own apart from the book as a whole.

Sullivan, Laurence E., ed. *Healing and Restoring: Health and Medicine in the World's Religious Traditions*. New York: Macmillan, 1989.
This book is the companion to Ronald Numbers and Darrel Amundsen, eds., *Caring and Curing* (Macmillan, 1986), a treatment of issues of health and medicine as they relate to religions in the Western world. This second volume, which can stand independently but is well read in tandem with the first, is involved with cultures, of both East and West, with which many readers may be less familiar. Among those presented are the Bantu-speaking peoples of Afric, Haitian devotees of Vodou, Buddhist traditions, Hindu traditions, Islamic tradition, Polynesian traditions, Native American and Mesoamerican traditions. A very helpful overview of information, as well as an opportunity for the reader to respect others while more deeply understanding herself, this book, like its companion, offers an overall description of women by their very absence. Depending upon a given essay, the reader may guess at the understanding of women in the tradition being addressed.

Tong, Rosemarie. *Feminist Thought: A Comprehensive Introduction*. Boulder, CO: Westview Press, 1989.
This work helps the reader to see varieties of feminist thinking, rather than to perceive or to use the word as an amorphous descriptor. Tong points out that feminist thought can be diverse - liberal, radical, psychoanalytic, socialist, existentialist, or postmodern. She limns the approaches of these by considering their differences in pursuing the "women questions." Considering the intersections of the both partial and provisional answers provided by the varieties of feminist thinking, Tong is able to show the lamentable aspects of women's oppression, as well as the ways in which so many women have triumphed, have encouraged one another, and have celebrated together, with regard to the challenges they have faced.

Vertinsky, Patricia. *The Eternally Wounded Woman: Women, Doctors and Exercise in the Late Nineteenth Century*. Manchester, England: Manchester University Press, 1990.

While this book does not intend to be primarily about descriptions of women, it does, in fact, highlight nineteenth century ones. A study of women, doctors, and exercise, accomplished by analyzing nineteenth century establishment medical reports and literary debates about women's physical attributes and social roles, it shows that much of medical discourse constituted women in a particular way. This was built upon descriptions of women powered primarily, if not solely, upon their generative function. Much of the discourse on female health, exercise, and sport, seen through biologically deterministic lenses, eventuated in medicalizing crucial female biological life events. The power of this book lies not only in its data and insights, but also in its relevance to a health care establishment which has not yet fully corrected these descriptions.

Weems, Renita J. *Just a Sister Away: A Womanist Revision of Women's Relationships in the Bible.* San Diego: LuraMedia, 1988.

Considering a number of biblical women and drawing insights and making analogies to contemporary women in ways relevant to Black women's experiences, Weems casts reflective light on women's interactions. Grounded in careful biblical scholarship but drawing connections to contemporary struggles, she encourages the reader to see old readings in a new way. Refreshing as well as helpful are the Questions for Thought at the end of each of Weems' nine stories. Inviting all women to new sharing, solidarity, and relating across boundaries, Weems can say, "We are frequently just a sister away from our healing."

Welch, Sharon D. *A Feminist Ethic of Risk.* Minneapolis, MN: Fortress Press, 1990.

Beginning with a discussion of the nuclear arms race, Welch presents a concern broader than that political issue. Her concern is over a "deep seated ethic of control" (p. 1). Ultimately, her book is interested in promises toward a transformative ethic which she calls an ethic of risk, and a theology of immanence, applicable to large ethical questions social and political crises. Emphasizing neither rights nor care as the basis of moral reasoning, Welch finds herself challenged by her experiences with African American women to criticize the presuppositions of Western moral theories. Her work complements both rights and care approaches to understandings of responsible action. In delineating an ethic of resistance and a feminist ethic of risk, Welch presents enlightening and empowering considerations upon the moral imagination. These, together with her thoughts on presence and solidarity, outline a demanding ethic, but one filled with the possibility of hope and joy in the work it calls forth.

CARE OF WOMEN

INTRODUCTION

This set of annotations is ultimately about women centered health care. In past times women's health was synonymous with gynecology, the assumption being that all other issues were treatable as men might be treated, since the male body and male experience was normative. Women centered health moves beyond woman as womb, or even woman as isolated body parts, to woman as whole person. It integrates gynecology as one aspect of the health concerns of woman as whole person in relationship. Thus, women centered concerns demand more permeable boundaries among medical specialties. Not only that, these concerns demand understanding of women's life cycle and whole health across the lifespan. They call for care for mind and body in relationship as well as life events, obligations, economics, and social location in relationship. For example, childhood sexual abuse may be seen later in PID, pelvic inflammatory disease, or PTSD, post-traumatic stress syndrome. Violence against women, recognized as a primary health issue for women, might be seen in a broader perspective, as underlying any number of "isolated" issues labeled as medical or psychological "pathologies," such as eating disorders, substance abuse, and chronic pain.

A health system, or at least a health approach for women as whole persons in relationship, would be involved in research on issues of specific importance to women's health, such as breast cancer and osteoporosis. It would call for basic science to explore sex-specific concerns, such as the place of estrogen in other than reproductive aspects. It would also be concerned about medical treatment and therapies based specifically on the actual physiology of women, rather than just assuming dosages and treatments which work for men. It would work at understanding women's lives in relationship so that some issues labeled pathological would be clearly seen as social constructs of who is woman, or social prescriptions for how women ought to act.

In the 1960s and 1970s women demanded knowledge of their own bodies and their own health issues. This movement opened the door to women's collaboration and cluster groups, women's demands for reproductive decision making, ownership of their bodies, their health, and their decision making on a more general level. Their push eventuated in changed birthing procedures, women's clinics, and more holistic health care. They organized for alternative practices, inclusion in research, and changes in medical curricula. In short, the women's health movement propelled the question of women's health from critique of the system, through growth in self-knowledge, to self-advocacy.

Women, both researchers and activists, helped health care systems to recognize that diseases common to both women and men, such as diabetes and heart disease, called for different treatment for women. They pointed out that specific health issues unique to women, and beyond reproductive ones, needed to be addressed. All the while, they had to uncover and deal with gender biases in diagnosis, in diagnostic taxonomies, and in research.

This topical section annotates books which concern women's overall health care, including considerations on religion and health. It also considers specific issues in women's health: cardiac concerns, violence against women, osteoporosis, breast cancer, and work-related problems for women. In attempting to mirror the integration which is part of care of women, I have chosen not to divide and label these specifics. Rather, I have simply listed all the books in alphabetical order by author, interweaving the concerns. Most titles will be fairly self-evident in terms of topics. A number of them will suggest companion readings further elucidating the same or a related topic. Many of the overall books include excellent chapters/essays which address these specific topics, and I have drawn out a few of these as a convenience to the reader. By the same token, diverse populations of women, such as African American women, Hispanic women, Asian women, and lesbian women, are included in chapters/essays of a good number of the books. Again, I annotate a few.

Some of the entries in these annotations fit clearly into the "Costs and Benefits" section. I have left them here not only as an indicator of the mutual intertwinement of the topics but also as an indicator of issues concerning women's overall health, specifically, poverty as a disease from which two out of three women worldwide suffer. The reader is pointed in further directions by the excellent references, bibliographies, and resources, such as organizations and clearinghouses, mentioned by many of the books included.

ANNOTATIONS

Achterberg, Jeanne. *Imagery in Healing: Shamanism and Modern Medicine.* Boston: Shambala, 1985.

Pointing out that imagery affects the body on many levels, Achterberg not only employs examples from the ordinary experience of most people but also traces they key role of imagery in medicine from the shaman to present studies in psychoneuroimmunology. In weaving the "golden thread" of imagery through the history of medicine, she not only presents a case for holistic medicine but also shows its implicit presence in a world of good science. The interdisciplinary character of the book weaves history, psychology, and science-social and behavioral as well as medical-in showing two basic ways that the image positively affects health. The first, Achterberg calls "preverbal" imagery, imagination acting upon one's own physical being by communicating with tissues, cells, and organs. The second she names "transpersonal," fleshing out the assumption that information can be transmitted from the consciousness of one person to the physical being of another. Clearly, the preverbal is more amenable to current scientific method. The transpersonal, validated more by qualitative types of data, is the bailiwick of theologians, philosophers, and medical historians.

ACT UP/New York Women and AIDS Book Group. *Women, AIDS, and Activism*. Boston: South End Press, 1990.

This book is the result of a collective and collaborative process. Its contributors represent a diversity of ethnicity, lifestyles, and health status. Its inclusion of the voices of HIV positive women and women with AIDS images the interconnection of care of women and care by women. Pointing out how little and how scattered is the information concerning women and HIV infection, the book offers information and modes of connection. It raises the challenges of changing research priorities, identifying and responding to women's treatment issues, demanding change in the health care system, and overcoming barriers to fighting HIV infection. Practical information on preventing HIV transmission, social and legal ramifications of HIV testing, and medical issues for women join questions of institutionalized racism, sexism, and heterosexism as topics presenting necessary information.

Alpert, Judith, ed. *Psychoanalysis and Women: Contemporary Reappraisals*. Hillsdale, NJ: The Analytic Press, 1986.

This book is divided into four sections: "Overview," "Freudian Theory and Beyond," "Female Patient," and "Female Analyst." In the twelve chapters subsumed under these divisions, the contributors consider controversies in female psychology. In this arrangement of sections and chapters, object relations models and self-psychology approaches are more prominent. The essay "Morality, Gender, and Analysis," by Judith Alpert and Jody Spencer, considers the theories of moral development of Freud, Horney, Kohlberg, and Gilligan with respect to gender differences. In reviewing Freud's belief that women have weaker superegos, the authors point out that he confuses values with observations. They review and criticize Kohlberg for creating the impression that women are deficient in moral reasoning. He does this by applying his work on cognitive development and moral measurement in males to women. Focusing on Gilligan's orientation toward attachment and connectedness, the authors consider her insight that men and women have distinct differences in values and moral development. Concluding by highlighting similarities and differences among the theorists being considered, Alpert and Spencer show these to have implications for clinical work.

Apple, Rima D., ed. *Women, Health and Medicine in America: A Historical Handbook.* New York: Garland, 1990.
This set of historical essays is a particularly helpful overview of the issues involved in care of women. Its contributors are generally well known for other contributions to the field of women and health. They cover issues as diverse as definitions of health, orthodox health care, alternative health care, social and political dynamics of women's health concerns, and considerations on health care providers. Because of its multifaceted character, parts of this book will be repeated in other sections of this annotated bibliography. Including a sectioned bibliography, this handbook points the reader in the direction of multiple paths of information.

Bair, Barbara, and Susan E. Cayleff. *Wings of Gauze: Women of Color and the Experience of Health and Illness.* Detroit, MI: Wayne State University Press, 1993.
This collection of essays portrays experiences of women of color, including African Americans, Latinas, Native Americans, and Southeast Asians. The editor notes early in the book that for women of color health is more than absence of disease or illness. Several of the contributors look at the folk healing which women of color practiced from the times of their early American heritage, customs which promoted an integrated well-being. The contributing scholars, often women of color themselves, address such topics as AIDS, alcohol and drug abuse, breast cancer, chronic illness, domestic violence, poverty, and prostitution. The essays also demonstrate how the effects of racist attitudes in helping agencies often result in lesser or no service to women of color. The narratives and histories of some of these experiences enable the reader to begin to

understand the struggle of these women to regain their health. The essays demonstrate that health for white American women is not necessarily health for others. Included are examples of efforts in various communities to provide the particular resources needed by women of color.

Benson, Herbert, M.D. *Timeless Healing: The Power and Biology of Belief.* New York: Scribner, 1996.

This book is the latest expression and set of implications of Benson's breakthrough publication *The Relaxation Response* (William Morrow & Co. 1975). Eminently readable, it invites personal reflection, as well as the reflection of the medical profession, upon the interrelationship of body, mind, and spirit. It is in some way representative of the more recent spate of books written by medical professionals recognizing a more holistic approach to the art of healing. Benson moves beyond dualism to tap the resources of brain and soul as he seeks to have mind/body medicine incorporated into faith and wellness, believing that biology is not separated from belief. Benson sees faith in a larger sense than organized religion, noticing that organized religion is easier to measure than belief. This book is well read in tandem with Jeanne Achterberg's *Imagery in Healing* (Shambala, 1985), the two being mutually enhancing.

Benson, Herbert, M.D., and Eileen M. Stuart, R.N., M.S. *The Wellness Book: The Comprehensive Guide to Maintaining Health and Treating Stress Related Illness.* New York: Birch Lane Press, 1992.

This book, a contribution to the emerging field of behavioral medicine as well as a practical approach to wellness education, provides the reader with a wide-ranging approach to health issues and an almost workbook convenience toward encouraging actual change. This result of twenty-five years of research as well as clinical practice at the Harvard Medical School and three of its five major teaching hospitals is eminently readable in both style and manageability of content. Page 6 provides a helpful "How to Use This Book" so that the reader knows immediately that each chapter will contain the objectives of the chapter, stories describing the experiences of patients, and a series of questions, exercises, or reflections.

Beyer, Marge, and Sunanda Ray. *Women and HIV/AIDS: An International Resource Book.* London: Pandora, 1993.

The value of this book lies in its unique approach for those interested in and/or concerned for women and HIV/AIDS issues. In bringing together material from a wide range of both published and unpublished resources, it provides a global view of both the problems and the potential in an area of health concerns growing progressively more important for women, yet still difficult to discuss. The book provides a guide to groups and resources which is not only concretely helpful to the reader but also apt to raise in the readers' minds ideas as to locating local resources. It also affords the opportunity for readers to contextualize their experience within a global picture, comparing and contrasting their own situation.

Blackburn, Clare. *Poverty and Health: Working with Families.* Philadelphia: Open University Press, 1991.

In concerning itself with the impact of poverty on health, this book considers, in particular, families with young children. Blackburn sets her context with a discussion on the meaning of poverty. In that context she is able to allude to measuring poverty, patterns of poverty, and causes of poverty. She takes notice that women's position, both from the standpoint of household/family responsibilities and from the point of view of economic status, leaves them particularly vulnerable to poverty. Though she does not state it, she is in agreement with those who see poverty as women's number one health issue on an international level. Blackburn shows poverty as a health hazard in terms of physiological, psychological, and behavioral processes through the lens of income as a health resource. In each of her chapters, she supplies not only an overarching context but also clear, concrete data and lucid "Conclusions and Implications for Practice."

Bruce, Judith, Mead Cain, and Daisy Hilse Dwyer. *A Home Divided: Women and Income in the Third World.* Stanford, CA: Stanford University Press, 1988.
A collection of articles which considers the issue of resource allocation within households, this book is not specifically focused on women's health. When one considers that, internationally, poverty and workload are the largest women's health issues, this volume offers a valuable introduction to the social and economic context within which many women struggle to sustain their well-being. Because the book places the question within Third World situations, the reader can draw the connections between First and Third World questions pertaining to women's well-being, which are more similar in some ways than one might expect, given cultural and economic stereotypes. At the same time one can see unique Third World considerations.

Brumberg, Joan Jacobs. *Fasting Girls: The Emergence of Anorexia Nervosa as a Modern Disease.* Cambridge, MA: Harvard University Press, 1988.
In this book, Brumberg considers anorexia nervosa as a complex response to a nexus of cultural messages around food, women's roles, body image, and family issues. In presenting this approach, Brumberg is primarily concerned with the rise of anorexia in the nineteenth and twentieth centuries. She disagrees with theories that the illness is related to a cultural ideal of female thinness or to girls' refusal of adult sexuality. In an afterword, the author focuses on the recurrence of anorexia from the 1960s onward, pointing toward it as an outcome of rapid change in society's approach to food and to sexuality. Brumberg sees the syndrome of anorexia nervosa as prevalent among hardworking and conscientious women whose expectations have been raised, but for whom there is not adequate social support. It is, in a sense, a secularized new perfectionism

that ties salvation to the achievement of an impossibly thin body. One practical implication is that Brumberg would like magazines to print fewer articles on weight loss and makeovers and more on a more whole social presentation of self.

Bullock, Susan. *Women and Work*. London: Zed Books, 1994.
This general introduction to global trends in women's work placesthe question within the broad framework of women and development, providing an overview of female labor and of women's initiatives to improve their plight. It considers factors which link women despite their enormously different experiences, while reporting on responses and initiatives by women and organizations from the local to the world level. The layout of the book is particularly inviting as it breaks down information into manageable segments with a pleasant and easily remembered format. Of particular interest is Chapter 6, "The Structures of Learning: Barrier or Key to the Door?" The aim of this work is full membership as persons in the human race for women as well as for men. It assumes that neither full development nor "gender symmetry" is yet achieved in the industrialized nations.

Buvinic, Mayra, and Sally W. Yudelman. *Women, Poverty and Progress in the Third World*. New York: The Foreign Policy Association, 1989.
Despite the gains since the International Women's Year Conference in Mexico City in 1975 and the United Nations Decade for Women, 1975-1985, the overall situation for women in developing and underdeveloped countries has not become appreciably better, and, in some cases, has grown worse. The authors take an updated look at these situations, pointing out the population link in terms of governments' ability to deliver vital services and to generate employment. Generally, economic contributions of women are still overlooked, especially their contribution of "invisible work." The authors find women's contributions all the more impressive since they have received such limited assistance not only from governments but also from international donor agencies.

Chapter 4, "Alleviating Women's Poverty: An Agenda for the 1990s," calls for providing women access to decently paid employment and productive resources, pointing out the larger outcome, given the links between women's work, family welfare, and sustainable growth. The authors consider education and health care as primary issues in alleviating women's poverty. Beyond that concern, one can consider poverty and low ascribed status as the number one international women's health issue.

Chavkin, Wendy, ed. *Double Exposure: Women's Health Hazards on the Job and at Home.* New York: Monthly Review Press, 1984.
This work is divided into three parts: "Women at Work," "Damned If You Do, Damned If You Don't: Work and Reproduction," "On the Homefront: Women at Home and in the Community." The section on "Women at Work" combines considerations on the electronic workplace, the health hazards of office work, the risks of the nursing profession, and the health problems of migrant and seasonal workers. The data, insights, and encouragements in both the preface and the introduction of this work are particularly helpful. While the issues discussed have become of greater conscious concern to larger publics in the 1990s, the publication date of the book points to longer years of awareness among groups of women. The profit of this work is enhanced for the reader by considering it in conjunction with *Office Work Can Be Dangerous to Your Health*, by Jeanne Stellman and Mary Sue Henifin (Pantheon, 1989).

Chodorow, Nancy. *Feminism and Psychoanalytic Theory.* New Haven, CT: Yale University Press, 1989.
This book shows the development of Chodorow's thought in integrating feminism and psychoanalysis. In Part I, "The Significance of Women's Mothering for Gender Personality and Gender Relations," writing from an object relations perspective, the author reviews her work on the construction of masculinity and femininity from the centrality of preoedipal questions. In Part II, "Gender, Self, and Social Theory," she

considers such issues as differentiation, gender differences, and intersubjectivity. In Part III, "Feminism, Femininity, and Freud," she points out the approaches to gender taken by psychoanalytic feminists and psychoanalysts. She encourages a beneficial continuing dialogue between psychoanalysts and feminists in the area of object relations. This encouragement is all the more important as the reader considers "Psychoanalytic Feminism and the Psychoanalytic Psychology of Women" in this same book. In this treatment, Chodorow shows the diversity of perspectives in psychoanalytic feminism and argues that these complex divisions make dialogue and ongoing communication difficult.

Cooper-White, Pamela. *The Cry of Tamar: Violence Against Women and the Church's Response.* Minneapolis, MN: Fortress Press, 1995.
An Episcopal priest, Pamela Cooper-White writes as woman, theologian, minister, and church leader. In placing before the reader incisive and insightful understandings and assessments of violence against women, Cooper-White places a challenge squarely before the eyes of the Christian churches. Prefacing her book with a reprise of the story of the rape of Tamar, the author presents Part I, "The Framework of Violence Against Women." Her considerations on power and modes of relationship set the stage for her second section, "Forms of Violence Against Women." It is this section which pertains most directly to care of women, in that it names, describes, and suggests practical responses to varying concrete forms of violence against women. Part III, "The Church's Response" appeals to ministers, as members of a healing profession, to develop, hone, and employ human and professional honesty, clarity, skill, and compassion. Cooper-White asks for nothing more than thoroughgoing change.

Corea, Gena. *The Hidden Malpractice: How American Medicine Mistreats Women.* New York: Harper Colophon, 1985.
This is a second edition, with afterword, of Corea's book originally

published in 1977. It considers the male dominance of the American health care system. Beginning with the historical exclusion of women from the medical professions and moving to the widespread mistreatment of women's health problems, Corea proposes solutions through women-controlled health care. The author attends to the dual role women play as health care receivers. They also serve as distributors of health care to spouse, children, and parents. She notes that women succumb to arteriosclerotic heart disease later in life than men do and that women's death rates after myocardial infarction are higher than those of men. This second edition makes the case that women's efforts to challenge the medical establishment since the time of Corea's first book have not reduced the malpractice against or mistreatment of women patients. This book is well read in conjunction with Karen Hicks' *Misdiagnosis: Woman as a Disease* (People's Medical Society, 1994).

Counts, Dorothy Ayers, Judith K. Brown, and Jaquelyn C. Campbell, eds. *Sanction and Sanctuary: Cultural Perspectives on the Beating of Wives.* Oxford, England: Westview Press, 1992.
Rich ethnographic descriptions showing the range and diversity of wife-battering around the world are a plus in this volume. While it gives a sense of the variation in the types and frequency of wife-battering, it provides information placing this abuse in the political, social, and economic context in which it occurs. It also presents findings on the relationship between battering and economic and political inequalities. The book provides three chapters dealing with theoretical contexts and fourteen cultural descriptions of wife-battering, presenting the reader with a broadened knowledge about varieties and commonalities among women with respect to this large health problem.

Crook, Marion. *My Body: Women Speak Out About Their Health Care.* New York: Insight Books/Plenum Press, 1995.
This book provides a look at women as they deal with the current doctor-centered health care systems in both Canada and the United

States. The author traveled to diverse areas of these countries to gather the experiences of women as they struggle to regain integrated, mind, body, and environmental health for themselves within the constraints of a male-dominated disease model of health care in both countries. Crook also examines how Canadian and United States systems can affect treatment or mistreatment, especially for poor women and for women living in non-urban areas. She discusses alternative types of care, both genuine and fraudulent. Through her interviews, the author discovered how women learn how to get information needed to make their own informed decisions, empowering and improving themselves in the process.

Dally, Ann G. *Women Under the Knife: A History of Surgery.* New York: Rutledge, 1991.
This work treats the question of appreciating advances in women's health obtained through gynecological practice, while being aware that these advances derived from men's exploitation of women through practices not inherently anti-woman but symptomatic of an unbalanced social contract between the profession of medicine and the patient. Dally, a practicing physician and psychiatrist, presents a history of obstetrics and gynecology which is a challenging study in the history of medicine. Her research provides a rational and scholarly piece of work. While Dally recognizes growth in women's articulation with regard to medical intervention, she points out the importance of understanding that the politics of medicine and medicine in politics are inseparable. Dally argues with the belief that whatever is convenient for the doctor must therefore be acceptable. She encourages in women a focused curiosity about their physical structure and body functions, a reminder repeated in a number of books from *Our Bodies, Ourselves* onward.

Dan, Alice J., ed. *Reframing Women's Health: Multidisciplinary Research and Practice.* Thousand Oaks, CA: Sage Publications, 1994.
This combination of practical as well as philosophical lenses through

which to view women's health brings together a distinguished group of contributors. It considers topics as diverse as gender inequity, exclusionary androcentric approaches to research, family medicine, international perspectives, domestic violence, lesbian health issues, reproductive questions, HIV, women's health scholarship, and women's health as a medical specialization. This work is indeed a sourcebook of current thought across disciplinary boundaries: medicine, nursing, psychology, social work, anthropolgy, women's studies, legal scholarship, and policy analysis. The fifteen recommendations made by Dan in her introduction, as well as the seven objectives stated under "What Next? Strategies to Achieve Excellence in Women's Health" in her epilogue, provide a clarity of understanding and a focus of direction, essential to bettering the situation of women and health. A beauty of this book is that it integrates academics and activism in such a manner that it can be read and enjoyed by professionals and nonprofessionals alike. Organized into six focused parts, this work contains chapters based upon material presented at a landmark conference in Chicago.

Davies, Miranda. *Women and Violence: Realities and Responses Worldwide.* London: Zed Books, 1994.
This collection of articles on women's efforts against violence presents very valuable international case studies. These studies not only raise key questions with regard to the causes of sexual violence, but also suggest effective ways of opposing it. The work is well read in conjunction with *Family Violence and Religion: An Interfaith Resource Guide* (Volcano Press, 1995) and Anna Kosof, *Battered Women: Living With the Enemy* (Franklin Watts, 1994).

Doyal, Lesley. *What Makes Women Sick.* New Brunswick, NJ: Rutgers University Press, 1995.
Very early in this book, Doyal states: "There is widespread belief that

doctors are the 'real' experts on women's health and that biomedicine holds the key to improving it. The book demonstrates the limitations of such an approach." Rather than exploring the interior of female bodies, Doyal's work steps into a larger realm to investigate the ways in which women's lives can make them sick. Through examining economic, social, and cultural influences on women's well-being, Doyal identifies the major obstacles that prevent women from having and sustaining optimal health. The author shows gender differences to be especially significant for women, since they usually mean inequality and discrimination. Though female subordination can take many forms, it is an extremely pervasive phenomenon, demonstrating endless variety as well as monotonous similarity. Doyal finds that men are usually dominant in the allocation of scarce resources and that this structured inequality has a major impact on women's health.

Ehrenreich, Barbara, and Deirdre English. *For Her Own Good: 150 Years of the Experts' Advice to Women.* Garden City, NY: Anchor Press/Doubleday, 1979.

In this examination of women and health care, the authors trace the professionalization of health care in the United States. They reassess advice from gynecologists, psychologists, psychoanalysts, and pediatricians, arguing that these experts usurped women's traditional healing skills and set themselves up as sole authorities. Later, male "experts," including media figures and popular writers, also imposed their ideas about proper female behavior, justifying their advice as a service to women for their own good. The authors point to a certain mystification of health care in the name of "scientific" guidance. Ultimately, they ask why women have been excluded from the policy and practice of medicine and what have been the consequences of this exclusion. Their presentation of the nineteenth century diagnosis of hysteria and their sketching of the scientific mystique lend an interesting spice to their work.

Ehrenreich, Barbara, and Deirdre English. *Witches, Midwives and Nurses: A History of Women Healers*. New York: Feminist Press, 1973.
Written from research and ideas used for their course on Women and Health at the State University of New York, both this book and its companion piece, *Complaints and Disorders: The Sexual Politics of Sickness* (Feminist Press, 1973), opened the way for a significant amount of research to follow in the late 1970s. In a style inviting a wide variety of readers, it presented a recovered history as well as logical and sociological critique. It pointed out the political, religious, and economic reasons for the veil that had fallen over women's place in healing, excluding them from leadership roles, and relegating them to subservient ones. Drawing a clear set of distinctions between professionalism and expertise, Ehrenreich and English encouraged women, especially those in the healing professions, to reclaim their story, challenge science by being aware of the monopoly of scientific knowledge, and open medicine to all women by breaking down the distinctions between women as health care workers and as health care consumers.

Ehrenreich, Barbara, Elizabeth Hess, and Gloria Jacobs. *Remaking Love: The Feminization of Sexuality*. Garden City, NY: Doubleday, 1986.
This book is a discussion of the "sexual revolution" of the 1960s and 1970s, especially its impact on ideas about female sexuality and sexual behavior. The authors analyze mainstream changes in attitudes, the role of popular culture figures, the influence of serious studies, and the reality of pornography. *Remaking Love* differs from many other analyses in its insistence that a women's sexual revolution actually occurred, fundamentally altering and expanding women's sexual potential.

Family Violence and Religion: An Interfaith Resource Guide, compiled by the Staff of Volcano Press. Volcano, CA: Volcano Press, 1995.
Written for clergy to become aware of and to learn how to help women escape family violence, this book defines forms of domestic violence.

Presenting myths and facts, it discusses abusers, women who are their partners, and some of the figures and factors in such relationships. There are chapters concerning cross-cultural and abusive relationships. The effect on children who live in such homes is presented, as well as considerations on the abuse and mistreatment of the elderly. The book addresses the responsibility of clergy in helping the victims and in speaking out against such abuse. Valuable for those who have little accurate knowledge of the subject, this book also addresses the religious concerns often raised by Christian women in abusive relationships and suggests strategies to challenge their misperceptions. Read in conjunction with Pamela Cooper-White's *The Cry of Tamar* (Fortress Press, 1995), this work offers guidance for the professional helper as well as the abused woman.

Felder, Raoul, and Barbara Victor. *Getting Away with Murder: Weapons for the War Against Domestic Violence.* New York: Simon and Schuster, 1996.

This look at the crime of domestic violence in America emphasizes that were the abuse of women in intimate relationships stranger abuse, the perpetrator would be immediately arrested and removed to jail. Instead, American society demands that the victim remove herself and her children and provides little in the way of protection and support. It discusses the difficulties in identifying not only the victims but also the abusers, and the ways society ignores this crime. Presenting examples of effective programs for batterers, and suggesting ways that the medical, legal/judicial, and social welfare systems must work together to make any headway in stopping this phenomenon, the book notes that when anyone part of the system fails a battered woman, she is left unprotected .

Firth-Cozens, Jenny, and Michael A. West. *Women at work: Psychological and Organizational Perspectives.* Philadelphia: Open University Press, 1991.

A current look at work issues for women in Britain, this book considers those issues which still indicate that the more things change the more they remain the same. Included are women's experiences not only in various fields but also at various levels of work, such as clerical, para-professional, managerial, and professional. The essays deal with the multiple issues involved for working women besides those posed directly by the work itself. The different working fields include the worlds of politics and technology. This work is well read in tandem with Ginny Nicarthy, Naomi Gottlieb, and Sandrah Hoffman's *You Don't Have to Take It* (Seal Press, 1993).

Fogel, Catherine Ingram, and Nancy Fugate Woods, eds. *Women's Health Care: A Comprehensive Handbook*. Thousand Oaks, CA: Sage Publications, 1995.
Particularly pertinent for this chapter are some chapters in Part I, especially those dealing with whole health across the lifespan; all of Part II; and Part IV dealing with individual health care issues for women. The contributors are women from interdisciplinary perspectives ranging from theoretical to clinical and practical expertises. Taking into consideration the political and social changes which women have experienced, this book not only analyzes women's health issues in sociological context but also points out the shift to personal proactivity and advocacy for women vis-à-vis their health care. The information is clear, detailed, and wide-ranging, and the references are fertile for further pursuit of the issues. This book is written in such a manner that it bridges what was once a gulf between women as health care providers and women as health care recipients.

Frankenhaueser, Marianne, Ulf Lundberg, and Margaret Chesney, eds. *Women, Work and Health: Stress and Opportunities*. New York: Plenum Press, 1991.
An international compendium of articles exploring the relationship between women's paid employment and their health. Four of the chapters or articles are particularly helpful since they provide overviews

of current research in important areas: Chapter 6 by Barnett and Marshall, "The Relationship Between Women's Work and Family Roles and Their Subjective Well-being and Psychological Distress," Chapter 8 by Haynes, "The Effect of Job Demands, Job Control and New Technologies on the Health of Employed Women: A Review," Chapter 2 by Waldron, "Effects of Labor Force Participation on Sex Differences in Mortality and Morbidity," and Chapter 4 by Kahn, "The Forms of Women's Work." The uniqueness of this last mentioned chapter is its attempt to come to a descriptive definition of work, upon which there is, as yet, no commonly agreed upon understanding.

Freeman, Jo, ed. *Women: A Feminist Perspective.* Palo Alto, CA: Mayfield, 1984.
This third edition of a helpful and multifaceted treatment of women's concerns offers important considerations concerning women's health. "Farewell to Alms: Women's Fate Under Welfare" by Diana Pearce traces the origins of welfare for women and children from poorhouses and orphanages to AFDC (Aid to Families with Dependent Children). Pearce sees women's poverty as quite different from men's because of the presence of their economically dependent children and because of gender handicaps in the arena of work. Pearce notices that the welfare system is based on a "male pauper model," with an emphasis on getting the recipient back into the workplace, and may be inappropriate for women with dependent children. There is no discussion of men's roles in creating and not providing for the dependent children. Also of note is "Poverty Is a Women's Problem" by Kathleen Shortridge. That essay discusses the predominance of women and children among the poor. While reviewing statistics, the author offers social explanations to counter the myth of female dependence on husbands and fathers. She proposes solutions, including preparing women for independent living.

Galbraith, Anna M. *Four Epochs of Woman's Life: A Study in Hygiene.* Philadelphia: W. B. Saunders and Company, 1901.

In her introduction, Galbraith ends with writing that the age of preventive medicine is upon American women, who, by educating themselves in regard to the "laws of nature which govern their physical being" will overcome the ignorance which causes so much suffering in their lives. The book instructs women in facts from puberty through menopause, and it encourages women to seek help from physicians throughout their life. Evident are many of the prevailing attitudes of the time, notwithstanding the fact that the author is a female physician. Perusing this book along with Christiana Northrup's *Women's Bodies, Women's Wisdom* (Bantam Books, 1995) affords the reader a clear contrast in styles and concerns across more than ninety years.

Germain, Adrienne, Judith Wasserheit, et al., eds. *Reproductive Tract Infections: Global Reports and Priorities for Women's Reproductive Health.* New York: Plenum Press, 1992.
This book includes clinical, epidemiological, social, and economic observations on reproductive tract infections and provides valuable case studies from a number of Third World countries. It points to women's powerlessness and invisibility when one considers that sexually transmitted diseases cause 750,000 women's deaths annually. That toll is more than AIDS in men, women, and children combined.

Giele, Janet, ed. *Women in the Middle Years.* New York: Wiley, 1982.
This book, produced through the work of a multidisciplinary study group, is a collection of papers on various demographic changes and sociological trends in women's health and their social and work roles. While it is written directly for professionals, it is readable with profit for nonprofessionals who are interested. Giele's paper, "Women in Adulthood: Unanswered Questions," reviews the literature on adult development, noting that male patterns are often viewed as the norm. She offers a model embracing aspects of both stage and life-span theory, a model which is multidimensional. The author points out that socially complex societies evidence more distinct stages of adult development,

while in societies with greater stability such distinct stages are not so discernible. In differentiating male from female development, Giele shows four major areas for research: the area of the physical, psychological issues, social roles, and institutional and cultural context.

Gilligan, Carol, Janie Victoria Ward, and Jill McLean Taylor, eds. *Mapping the Moral Domain.* Cambridge, MA: Harvard University Press, 1988.

This collection of essays is well read in conjunction with new medical curricula. The themes of developmental reconsiderations are echoed in later plans to educate for women's whole health across the lifespan, such as the COGME Report. Of particular benefit are the essays such as 5 and 10 considering moral sensibilities in adolescents, combined with new perspectives on self roles and relationships. The essays considering mothers, physicians and lawyers are natural additions to the new discussions of developmental issues in girls These are essays 11, 12, and 13. In all the contributions to this book the writers raise prime questions, saving the reader from gathering such diversity from any number of other books.

Graham, Hilary. *Hardship and Health in Women's Lives.* New York: Harvester Wheatsheaf, 1993.

A look at the recent statistics and experiences of the 6.4 million women in Britain who live with and care for children, usually their own, under the age of sixteen. The book examines the ever-increasing hardships in those women's lives as the number of families in Britain continues to grow amid economic, social, political, and cultural difficulties which adversely affect the health of such women who are poorer and poorer. The author uses personal anecdotes of the women involved in the struggle to take care of the children and themselves.

Guide to Clinical Preventive Services, second edition. Report of the U.S. Preventive Services Task Force. Baltimore: Williams and Wilkins, 1996.

A cooperative venture between the U.S. and Canadian Task Forces, as well as between the federal government and the private sector, produced the first edition of the *Guide to Clinical Preventive Services*, reviewing evidence for over 100 interventions. The second edition has reevaluated each preventive service, with each chapter rewritten and 11 new chapters added. Written primarily for primary care clinicians, other allied health professionals, and students, it is readable for others who are interested. Its usefulness to the general reader lies in several issues: understanding sifting processes in health care management, noticing the move to primary care, seeing prevention as a health care value, and encountering specific information on concrete physical conditions.

Haas, Ann Pollinger. "Lesbian Health Issues: An Overview." In Alice J. Dan, ed., *Reframing Women's Health: Multidisciplinary Research and Practice*. Thousand Oaks, CA: Sage Publications, 1994.
Providing excellent resources and references, this essay addresses the question of whether and how lesbians health issues are different from those of any other women. The author considers the background of the questions as well as lesbians' interactions with health care professionals. She addresses the physical health status of lesbians, including specific health issues such as cancer, sexually transmitted diseases, menopause and aging, and mental health, along with legal and partnership concerns. Her "Strategies for Improving Lesbian Health and Health Care" are particularly helpful and practical.

Harland, Marion. *Eve's Daughters, or Common Sense for Maid, Wife, and Mother*. New York: Charles Scribner's Sons, 1885.
An early attempt to educate women regarding their human nature, refuting some of the common attitudes and societal practices at the end of the nineteenth century in America. Especially noteworthy is the author's advocacy of even higher education of young women, even as she cautions against some of the then current beliefs about women's health, most particularly, those regarding the balancing of mental and physical

work. Additionally the reader will discover various yet typical attitudes about a number of aspects of middle American life.

Hartman, Betsy. *Reproductive Rights and Wrongs: The Global Politics of Population Control and Contraceptive Choice*. New York: Harper and Row, 1987.

Exploring the relationship between population control and reproductive choice in the Third World, this book puts population problems and population policies into a wider social and economic framework in order to assess whole health and family planning programs which might better meet the needs of the poor. Analyzing international issues surrounding population control and reproduction, emphasizing the importance of choice and "the inviolability of individual reproductive rights," Hartman argues that, since improved living conditions and changes in the position of women lead to smaller families, basic social and economic changes in developing countries will reduce population problems and eliminate need for Western imposition of technology-oriented solutions. Individual chapters examine international organizations promoting population control and controversies over various methods of contraception. An appendix lists organizations involved in global reproductive issues. This book is well read in conjunction with Ruth Dixon-Mueller's *Population Policy and Women's Rights* (Praeger, 1993).

Hays, Hoffman R. *The Dangerous Sex: The Myth of Feminine Evil.* New York: G. P. Putnam's Sons, 1964.

This book presents a social history of women as less than men in Western society throughout various historical ages. It draws on some examples from literature in its aim to demonstrate that the literary is a reflection of the beliefs and attitudes of a particular time, in this case, beliefs and attitudes of men toward women. The author states his opinion that society has reached a crisis in the relationships between women and men, that men must give up their "magical attitude toward the second sex" if things are to improve.

Kosof, Anna. *Battered Women: Living with the Enemy.* New York: Franklin Watts, 1994.

A short volume which presents the background of domestic violence and examines major myths, behavior, and facts in the stories of several women which illustrate various aspects in the cycle of violence in intimate relationships. Kosof also describes what happens when women attempt to leave such situations, and how the police and courts often ignore or refuse to enforce laws which could hold the abuser accountable for the behavior and begin to break abusive patterns. She describes the importance of shelters as safe places for abused women as they receive the support they need to gain the strength to change their own lives. The book concludes by emphasizing that American society must confront the extent of family abuse and recognize that it is not a woman's issue but a human issue. Several appendices provide quick looks at myths, along with statistics, and checklists to recognize abuse and possible abusers. Written for high schools, it is good for anyone who wants easy-to-read information on this topic.

Kurth, Ann, ed. *Until the Cure: Caring for Women with HIV.* London: Yale University Press, 1993.

This book is well read in conjunction with Marge Beyer and Sunanda Ray, *Women and HIV/AIDS: An International Resource Book* (Pandora, 1993), and ACT UP (New York Women and AIDS Book Group) *Women, AIDS, and Activism* (South End Press, 1990). Based as it is on U.S. experience, containing often   succinct   and valuable information, this U.S. reference book has importance for working "hands on" with women living with HIV disease. It presents a picture of useful practice in helping women to cope with HIV in the absence of a cure. This book can be read with equal benefit by pastors and health care workers.

Legato, Marianne, M.D., and Carol Colman. *The Female Heart: The Truth About Women and Coronary Artery Disease.* New York: Simon and Schuster, 1991.

Having both experienced, through people in relationship to them, the results of women's heart problems neither being taken as seriously as men's nor being treated as aggressively, the authors chose to write this book. Beliefs still held by many men and women, physicians and lay alike, that heart attacks are a health problem for men, continue in part because the majority of cardiac research has been focused on men. These beliefs and research priorities have not encouraged women's education to their own heart care and their own attention to symptoms. Beginning with Chapter 1, "The Normal Female Heart and How It Works," Legato and Colman present helpful, detailed, and readable data on anatomy and on women's specific heart issues. This book is not about biology only. Dealing with the whole woman, it proceeds to discussion of women at risk for heart attacks as well as body-mind approaches to wellness. It provides useful and supportive information on dealing with coronary artery disease as well as modes of preventive and proactive care. This work contains a section on resources as well as a selected bibliography.

Leonard, Ann. *Seeds 2: Supporting Women's Work Around the World.* New York: The Feminist Press, 1995.

With an introduction by Martha Chen and afterwords by Mayra Buvinic, Misrak Elias, Rounaq Jahan, Caroline Moser, and Kathleen Staudt, this collection of essays is part of a series commissioning and publishing women-focused case studies of economic development projects. The increasing feminization of poverty disappointed the hopes of some that by the end of the United Nations Decade for Women, 1975-1985, efforts such as *Seeds* might have become unnecessary. The first Seeds study, *Seeds, Supporting Women's Work in the Third World* published by The Feminist Press, 1989 consisted of nine case studies and four essays. The seven new case studies in this book illustrate change in the direction of moving to broaden the concept of women's work from simply earning income to generating livelihoods and improving economic status, and moving to integrate women into various sectors of social and economic development. Both of these are issues which are ultimately prime to women's health. *Seeds 2* shows strategies pointed toward increasing women's access to land, labor, and credit markets; providing health care, child care, and other support services; and organizing women for collective action and political participation. This collection places emphases on health and education, more appropriate and beneficial land use, and better attention to ecology.

Luker, Kristin. *Abortion and the Politics of Motherhood.* Berkeley: University of California Press, 1984.

This major study of the pro-choice and antiabortion movements in the United States intended to illuminate specific issues concerning abortion. At the same time, Luker's detailed examination of motivations, attitudes, goals, and organizational techniques of committed activists provided insight into women's roles in political movements and advocacy. Beginning with the history of the issue in the United States, Luker traces the emergence of abortion as the subject of political debate and follows the development of oppositional movements. She analyzes the world-view and commitments of activists on both sides and places the positions in larger political, philosophical, and religious contexts. Through personal interviews with activists, Luker makes the case that deeply involved activists oversimplify public opinion. Placing the debate in the cultural context of attitudes toward motherhood, Luker notices that anti-abortionists place the biological (reproductive) before the social (women as paid workers). The author includes considerations of political strategies and futures of the movements.

McGoon, Michael D., ed. *Mayo Clinic Heart Book.* New York: William Morrow and Company, 1993.

While this book presents clearly written and readable general information, it still seems to assume that heart issues are male issues. The only direct treatment in terms of care of women is the information contained in the final six pages of text. That six-page consideration is titled "Women and Heart Disease" and is subsumed under Part VI, "Issues in Cardiology." The book remains a good example of continuing belief systems, imaging by scope and placement, how women and coronary artery disease are still treated in some spheres.

McLeod, Eileen. *Women's Experience of Feminist Therapy and Counseling*. Buckingham, England: Open University Press, 1994.

Noticing a dearth of material from the viewpoint of women who are the beneficiaries of feminist therapy, the author takes these beneficiaries as a distinct focus of and contribution to this book. She draws on the experiences and views of such women with regard to the help and drawbacks they found in feminist therapy and counseling. The sample of women represented in the book is those who attended a provisional feminist therapy and counseling center in Britain during its first two years of operation. Each chapter discusses the limitations of analyzing solely in terms of subordination through gender, how egalitarian are the theories therapists and counselors employ, and how egalitarian are the outcomes. McLeod makes the case that taking account of women's diversity is essential, that feminist therapy is helpful only to the extent that it offers an experience of relative freedom from subordination, and that initiatives beyond therapy, including dealing with a range of social inequalities, are also essential to realizing women's emotional well being.

Mahowald, Mary Briody. *Women and Children in Health Care: An Unequal Majority*. New York: Oxford University Press, 1993.

This work deals primarily with reproductive, fetal, and neonatal issues in women's lives. After discussing aspects of a more egalitarian physician-patient relationship, the author deals with such issues as fertility, abortion, in vitro development, treatment of viable fetuses, and fetal tissue transplantation. The rights to make decisions regarding disabled newborns, as well as children's rights in the decision-making process regarding their own potentially terminal illnesses, are also discussed. Paying attention to the effect that the feminization of poverty has on women, on children, and on the elderly, the author ends with a discussion of a just care-based decision-making process which would empower women who are currently powerless in many medical decisions and situations.

Matteo, Sherri, ed. *American Women in the Nineties: Today's Critical Issues.* Boston: Northeastern University Press, 1993.

This collection reiterates the connection between the stress of inequality and questions of health. The book focuses on education, employment policies and practices, and the resulting economic consequences which can greatly affect a woman's health. Other more directly connected topics include health insurance, AIDS, abortion, and sexual harassment. Lastly, the book focuses on politics and political thinking, areas where more female participation is critical in order to effect policy change and practice. The book includes excerpts from *How Schools Shortchange Girls*, the American Association of University Women 1992 report which reviewed research revealing the power differential in the American educational system, a reality which ultimately deprives at least half of our children of their full potential as mature individuals, workers, citizens, and parents.

Miner, Valerie, and Helen E. Longino, eds. *Competition: A Feminist Taboo?* New York: The Feminist Press, 1987.

Prior to contemporary feminism, prime public settings for competition did not welcome women. Rather, competition among women defined for them competition as a whole. Women might compete with attributes other than beauty, and for prizes other than men, primarily in women's schools and colleges. With feminism and the civil rights movement came widening opportunities. At the same time, feminists were considering the need to replace competition with collaboration. This book seeks to look at competition as a double-edged sword. From those who purvey a sense of not-good-enough to others in order to eliminate competition against themselves, competition is a tool to maintain the *status quo ante*. For others who see the not-good-enough person also as a threat, there may be a need to eliminate the other from competition. The lack of self-confidence which can engender senseless competition at the same time makes collaboration difficult. Thus, lack of self-confidence sours both competition and collaboration. This book points toward the reality that healthy competition brings experience and strength. It breaks the silence over contemporary competition among women, presenting essays with varying conceptual, experiential, and analytic points of view. In setting forth the intersections between competition and collaboration, these essays raise questions concerning the differences among striving for excellence, striving for control, and striving for success. This book may offer women in the healing professions some important reflections as they strive for both equity and caring collaboration.

Mirsky, Judith, ed. *Private Decisions, Public Debate: Women, Reproduction and Population.* London: Panos London, 1994.
This collection of case studies was published in preparation for the 1994 International Conference on Population and Development in Cairo, Egypt, in order to "focus on solutions to accelerating population growth and deepening impoverishment particularly affecting developing countries." The essays deal with a variety of current health issues in developing countries including son preference, religion, untreated sexually transmitted disease, female genital mutilation, and AIDS. The essays not only focus on the everyday realities and the human costs connected with these issues but also recognize the much larger issues involved for society and government. The authors see that tending to these issues can eventually provide that women will have a status and choice equal to those of men, thus improving women's quality of life.

Muller, Charlotte F. *Health Care and Gender.* New York: Russell Sage Foundation, 1990.

This book studies the results of many studies regarding differences in health care. It examines these differences between women and men, black women and white women, and men of diverse economic, marital, or parental status. The statistics, fairly current at the time of this work's publication, still paint a dismal picture for women and their health care in the United States. Though some of the studies were ten or more years old, they present accurate representations of present results. The author, in discussing some of the studies, points out flaws and indicates how the failure to ask pertinent questions resulted in less than useful information. This work is well read in tandem with Helen B. Holmes and Laura M. Purdy, *Feminist Perspectives in Medical Ethics* (Indiana University Press, 1992), and Susan Sherwin, *No Longer Patient* (Temple University Press, 1992).

Nechas, Eileen, and Denise Foley. *Unequal Treatment: What You Don't Know About How Women Are Mistreated by the Medical Community.* New York: Simon & Schuster, 1994.

In 1986, the National Institute of Health mandated that women, who were left out of medical research, were to be included in the study populations of grant proposals, unless there were telling scientific reasons for their exclusion. Four years later it was found that the mandate was still being ignored. This book deals with the many ways women are ignored in all aspects of medicine, whether as part of research populations, as physicians, as researchers, or, most especially, as patients. There are chapters which discuss the effects of such neglect and ignorance on the health of women with regard to specific topics, including heart disease, breast cancer, AIDS, psychological concerns, aging, poverty, and maternity issues. The author ends with a chapter on how women are beginning to be seen, to be heard, and to work vis-à-vis this unequal treatment.

Northrup, Christiane, M.D. "Menopause." In *Women's Bodies, Women's Wisdom.* New York: Bantam Books, 1995.

Northrup begins her discussion of menopause with considerations upon our cultural inheritance. She deals with hormones, fear of aging, types of menopause, and symptoms of menopause. Her approach is one eminently respectful to the reader, providing information and experience, but leaving decisions to the reader. Weaving spirituality and sensible sifting through her presentation, she maintains a holistic approach. Northrup presents considerations on natural menopause and phytoestrogens (natural hormones in food) as well as artificial menopause and synthetic estrogen replacement therapy. Particularly helpful to some readers are the pages on osteoporosis. The presentation is clear and the information direct. The author looks at screening methods for bone density as well as nutritional and exercise approaches for bone health. In her treatment of mood swings and depression, she considers the experience of "fuzzy thinking." She also provides discussions of ERT (estrogen replacement therapy), breast cancer, and heart disease, all particularly pertinent to menopause. Perhaps most practically helpful to the reader is the material included under her subheading "Self Care During Menopause."

Oakley, Ann. *Essays on Women, Medicine and Health*. Edinburgh: Edinburgh University Press, 1993.
A collection of essays, lectures, and papers written between 1981 and 1992, this book is an integration of perspectives from social science, history, literature, and experience, all of which are held together by themes. These themes are represented by the overall concerns of the book's sections: divisions of labor, motherhood, technology, and methodology. Within those themes, the author considers some problems of the medical profession, issues around birthing, and comparison of research models. Because the multidisciplinary approaches are so well interwoven, this book provides the reader a helpful "feel" for the context as well as the concrete questions of women's health.

Royston, Erica, and Sue Armstrong. *Preventing Maternal Deaths.* Geneva: WHO, 1989.

This is a monograph produced under the auspices of the World Health Organization as part of its campaign against maternal mortality. It provides a clear and comprehensive overview of the causes and consequences of morbidity and mortality during childbearing and discusses possible solutions.

"Screening for Postmenopausal Osteoporosis." In *Guide to Clinical Preventive Services*, second edition. Report of the U.S. Preventive Services Task Force. Baltimore: Williams and Wilkins, 1996.

Stating that about 70% of fractures in persons aged 45 or older are types that are related to osteoporosis and that most of these injuries occur in postmenopausal women, this entry reminds the reader that low bone density is associated with an increased rate of fracture. The principal risk factors for osteoporosis are listed: female sex, advanced age, Caucasian race, low body weight, and bilateral oophorectomy before menopause. Smoking is a probable risk for hip fracture, but it is a less reliable predictor of bone mass. The entry considers accuracy of screening tests as well as whether screening is recommended and/or effective at present. It notes that both costs and inconvenience of screening do not recommend it. Further research is needed to estimate clinical effectiveness as well as cost effectiveness of such screening. This entry does, however, recommend counseling as to universal prevention measures.

Sidel, Ruth. *Keeping Women and Children Last: America's War on the Poor.* New York: Penguin Books, 1996.

This book is a sequel to *Women and Children Last: The Plight of Poor Women in Affluent America*, which re-examines poverty in America. The author argues that, since the Cold War has subsided, women in poverty have become the enemy. She discusses and illustrates how "American society has not adjusted to contemporary family patterns, to current economic realities, and continues racial, gender, and class inequities" (p. 49). As a result women are blamed and children become the real victims. After listing myths, the author cites recent statistics and notes that because of use of an almost forty-year-old formula for calculating the poverty line, the number of people calculated as living in poverty is artificially low, compared to any realistic method of calculating living expenses. In fact, "dependent aid to corporations," or "corporate welfare," is in no danger of being dismantled in the way the federal government is currently attempting to dismantle the welfare system.

Smith, John M. *Women and Doctors: A Physician's Explosive Account of Women's Medical Treatment and Mistreatment in America Today.* New York: Dell, 1993.

A fellow of the American College of Obstetricians and Gynecologists, Smith offers the reader stories of incompetence, disrespect, and irresponsibility with regard to gynecological treatment of women. Questioning whether it is inappropriate for men to be gynecologists, Smith claims that a male cannot fully understand a female patient's problems. Perhaps the most direct help of this book comes from the author's provision of practical guides for detecting an untrustworthy doctor and his presentation of questions which a patient ought to ask her doctor. He offers a helpful section covering the most common gynecological problems and outlining treatment options. He calls for an informed and empowered female patient and encourages the entrance of more women into the field.

Spain, Daphne, and Suzanne M. Bianchi. *Balancing Act: Motherhood, Marriage and Employment Among American Women.* New York: Russell Sage Foundation, 1996.

A revision of *American Women in Transition* (1986). this work presents choices facing women as they balance these three areas of their lives in the latter part of the twentieth century. It discusses progress and regression in various areas, noting that the authors believe that the wage gap has narrowed enough so that "slow, steady progress toward equality is being made." Especially interesting is the demographic information showing the great changes that have occurred regarding motherhood and marriage. This book presents statistics for black, Hispanic, and white women, with comparisons to other Western industrialized nations when possible.

Statman, Jan Berliner. *The Battered Woman's Survival Guide.* Dallas: Taylor, 1990.
A short, easy-to-read book written at the time when Battered Woman's Syndrome was the explanation for women's behavior. The author gives a multi-page list of warning questions to help discern a potential batterer but the result is that, in truth, you can't tell what a batterer will look or sound like until it's too late. Four cases histories, none of which resulted in the woman's death, are presented. However, one of the wives in these case histories, a woman who killed her battering husband, was convicted of murder. Unfortunately for some, the book can easily lead the reader to believe that if she stays within the system, the police and the law will be able to help her.

Stellman, Jeanne, and Mary Sue Henifin. *Office Work Can Be Dangerous to Your Health.* New York: Pantheon, 1989.
The book, a study of health risks to office workers, includes data on faulty or badly designed equipment, careless office design and furniture arrangement, and inadequate safety provisions. This edition reviews and updates an earlier one published in 1983. The 1989 version provides a useful summary of current information on the hazards of office work and reads very well in conjunction with several essays in *Women, Work and Health* (Plenum Press, 1991) edited by Marianne Frankenhaeuser, Ulf Lundberg, and Margaret Chesney, such as "Health Effects of Clerical Employment" and "Health Effects of VDT Work." There is profit to the

reader in looking at Wendy Chapkin, ed., *Double Exposure: Women's Health Hazards on the Job and at Home* (Monthly Review Press, 1984).

Stepanich, Kisma K. *Sister Moon Lodge: The Power and Mystery of Menstruation.* St. Paul, MN: Llewellyn Publications, 1993.

An easily readable volume which encourages women to tap into the power and mystery of menstruation throughout their lives, by discovering some Native American women's practices and wisdom. The author provides stories of practices, creative writing, ritual, and custom to help women discover the power that lies within themselves because they experience menarche, menstruation, and menopause. She also provides knowledge of herbal remedies for relief of symptoms and encourages the use of space within for journaling of the readers' own experiences.

Todd, Alexandra Dundas. *Intimate Adversaries: Cultural Conflicts Between Doctors and Women Patients.* Philadelphia: University of Pennsylvania Press, 1989.

This two and one-half year study of audio taped and observed interactions between male gynecologists and female patients in a private practitioner's office and in a community clinic uses sociolinguistic methods to study the way male doctors and female patients communicate. Todd found that while male doctors concentrate on a biomedical approach to the body or organ, the patients embed their concerns in broader contextual experiences based upon their specific lives and relationships. Thus, often, in medical encounters, what the patient needed to address was ignored. While Todd saw this gap in doctor and patient perspectives as having three specific patterns, they boil down, in one way or another, to who is perceived to have power in the conversation. Generally, "women's talk," framed in life and social context, is considered less important.

United Nations. *Violence Against Women in the Family.* Vienna: Center
for Social Development and Humanitarian Affairs, 1989.
The first international summary of information on domestic violence
against women, this study discusses the volume, the results, and the
causes of violence against women in their own homes. Most helpful to
the reader is the naming and examination of a range of possible
responses to this important women's health issue. For readers in the
United States, where domestic violence is cause for the largest
percentage of women's visits to hospital emergency rooms, this volume
is particularly pertinent. Its presentation of alternatives encourages
readers to develop responses from the perspective of the situational
context in which they find themselves.

White, Evelyn C., ed. *The Black Women's Health Book: Speaking for
Ourselves.* Seattle: Seal Press, 1990.
This edition presents a broad range of black female experiences and
insights related to health approached from multifaceted perspectives.
Mirroring a diversity of disciplines and dimensions, this creative tapestry
presents a full and nuanced picture of the wisdom, caring, insight,
resiliency, and determination of black women as they tend their health,
support one another, and face the inequities of the health care system by
speaking for themselves. The roster of contributors includes health care
providers and activists, historians, literary women, journalists, artists,
educators, ministers, and storytellers. Many of their names will be
immediately recognizable to the reader.

Wilkinson, Sue, and Celia Kitzinger, eds. *Women and Health: Feminist
Perspectives.* London: Taylor & Francis, 1994.
Concerned that a good deal of the work on women's health has
remained within disciplinary boundaries, the editors developed their
project into a multidisciplinary contribution with a feminist focus. The
individual authors in this collection of essays are British, and they reflect
on broader international differences where appropriate. Rather than

placing emphasis on women's traditional roles, reproductive ones in particular, these contributors consider the issues surrounding women's health and well-being across a span of activities and life stages. Chapter 3, concerning pregnancy and body image; Chapter 5, concerning waged work and women's well-being; and Chapters 6 and 7, concerning substance abuse, are particularly useful for their data as well as their reframing of the questions.

CARE BY WOMEN

INTRODUCTION

Given new epistemologies, both those created by women, from the consciousness raising and health study groups of the 1960s, through the more academically articulate methodologies for feminist theologies, feminist histories, feminist medical ethics, and feminist sociological theories, given the interconnected world-views afforded by quantum mechanics, it is difficult if not impossible to separate care of women and care by women. Both find their roots in interwoven relationships.

Based upon these notions, this section presents annotations involving the history of women in the healing professions, life concerns of women in the healing professions, information about, by, and for women who are called upon for health care but are not considered to be members of the healing professions, as well as concerns of women cared for by women. Some entries are placed here because of the outstanding research or reflective contribution made by women redounding to the care of women. A number of these will pertain to healing professions other than those which the reader may be accustomed to seeing as healing professions, such as education, ministry, and social work. Ultimately, this section considers women who are commonly understood to be in the health care professions as well as those in healing professions not labeled as health care professions but still pertinent to women's whole health.

In the highly visible, public, and professional arena of health care women outnumber men by a three to one ratio. They are, however, clustered in the situations of lower pay, less prestige, and less autonomy. They tend to be primarily assistants and technicians. Nurses and aides constitute 90% of women in professional health care employment. Invisible and unpaid, in the

United States, for example, is "Dr. Mom," the target of marketing aimed at her responsibility for the health of her family. Even in two-income families, women do the largest percentage of homekeeping and of caretaking. Traditional expectations of mothers, daughters, and daughters-in-law still function as women provide 80-90% of unpaid health care in the United States. In terms of changed actuarial tables resulting from longer life expectancies, that "women's work" which is unpaid health care has increased. Women in the sandwich generation, those who are tending to the health of their parents as well as of their children, are the overwhelmingly large percentage of those who care for elder and disabled family members. They are also called upon to care for those relations currently discharged from hospitals "quicker and sicker" due to diagnostic related groups which limit hospital stay. While the financial reports of the health care system might show that this mode of home care is less expensive, it is hardly less expensive to the unpaid women involved in caretaking, not only to their purse but also to their health. In some sense, the issue of care by women is microcosmic of the world at large and its gender issues. Women do the greatest percentage of the work but have the least status and the smallest percentage of ownership.

Women have also been, and are, community activists, environmental activists, and alternative health care providers. They have effectively changed professional definitions of health, encouraging new emphases upon the art of health care, calling for greater self-education and self-help, in effect placing decisions concerning any woman's body back into the hands of its owner.

Because the healing professions are far wider than the publicly recognized health care professions, I have included the caring work of and pertinent considerations with regard to educators and ministers as well as doctors, nurses, social workers, massage therapists, and other therapeutic professionals. While most of the books concerning spirituality are placed in the section, "Addictions", several are placed here as an indication of one of the breakthrough ways in which women have cared for women. As the health system has become progressively aware of the place of spirituality in healing, including physical health, women's contribution, both practical and experiential, as well as published, ought to be recognized.

A number of the books in this set of annotations contain the stories of women in the healing professions, such as the works of Walsh, Morantz-Sanchez, Achterberg, Abram, and Melosh. For the readers' convenience, I annotate a few of those chapters. Others, like *Stress and the Woman Physician, Despite the Odds,* and *Strangers in the Sacred Grove,* address issues pertinent to women healers. Much of the material in "Care of Women" could also be situated in the current chapter given the groundbreaking research as well as the interrelationships and multiple roles of women. The two sections could be read as one.

ANNOTATIONS

Abram, Ruth J., ed. *"Send Us a Lady Physician": Women Doctors in America, 1835-1920.* New York: W. W. Norton and Company, 1985. A collection of essays, this work explores in greater detail some of the ideas presented in Barbara Ehrenreich and Deirdre English, *Witches, Midwives and Nurses* (Feminist Press, 1973). The essays present the professionalization of medicine in the nineteenth century United States, women's entrance into the medical profession, and the reason for the decline in the percentage of women physicians at the end of the nineteenth century. The beauty of this text is not only that it presents information well worth recapturing but also that it is arranged in discrete, enjoyable to read pieces and peppered with enlightening pictures and timelines. These not only clarify information but also give a felt sense of the data involved. Of particular interest to the reader concerned with women and health might be the following three essays: "Will There Be a Monument?: Six Pioneer Women Doctors" by Ruth J. Abram, "Co-Laborers in the Work of the Lord: Nineteenth Century Black Women Physicians" by Darlene Clark Hine, and "Every Woman Is a Nurse: Work and Gender in the Emergence of Nursing" by Barbara Melosh. The reader who enjoys this history will be well served in perusing Mary

Roth Walsh, *"Doctors Wanted: No Women Need Apply,"* (Yale University Press, 1977), and Barbara Melosh, *"The Physician's Hand":* *Work Culture and Conflict in American Nursing* (Temple University Press, 1982).

Achterberg, Jeanne. *Woman as Healer.* Boston: Shambala, 1990.

This work is divided into four parts: "Medicine Woman: The Ancient Cosmic Connection," "Women and the Genesis of Scientific Thought," "Women and the Professionalization of the Healing Arts," "Twentieth Century Women and the State of the Healing Arts and Sciences." It is a historical approach recognizing women's contributions to the healing professions. While it helps for an understanding of how and why women have arrived at their present situation, it points at possibilities for improving the situation, eliciting a return to concepts of caring in the art of curing. The author's section on midwifery and her considerations on female physicians of the nineteenth century encourage a reclamation of women's story at the same time that they evoke critical thought. The sweep and dynamic of the historical presentation makes this work easy and enjoyable to read. Particularly interesting is the presentation on "The Healer and the Healing System" and the diagram of an interconnected web in Chapter 17, "Life in the Balance."

Ainley, Marianne Gosztonyi, ed. *Despite the Odds: Essays on Canadian Women and Science.* Montreal: Vehicule Press, 1990.

The essays in this collection address the lack of visibility which has been women's lot in the scientific community. The author considers in particular the Canadian scientific community. Historically blocked from higher education, obstructed from upward career mobility, and under-represented in historical accounts of scientific achievements, women in positions of institutional decision-making power in the scientific community have been a disproportionately low percentage of the total number of those women involved in the scientific enterprise. The contributors to this edition point out the activities and accomplishments of Canadian women scientists. They bring to light accomplishments and difficulties of these women. This book represents a wide range of scientific pursuits: medicine, mathematics, technology, social science, and applied science. It is a work not only of women's history but also of the history of science in Canada.

American Medical Association, Women in Medicine Services. *Women in Medicine in America: In the Mainstream.* Chicago, IL: American Medical Association, 1991.
The Women in Medicine Services of the AMA, American Medical Association, attends to continuing information concerning women physicians. This report, including statistical tables representing stages of a female physician's career, discusses the issues facing women in medicine. The first section provides data about the history of women in medicine. The second section considers the years of training, including residency. It also attends to questions around combining work and family, role models, gender inequities, child care and maternity leave, and choice of specialty. The third section concerns itself with women and practice. It includes tables on specialty and board certification, marital status and children, academic medicine, weeks worked per year, and income. Concluding that medicine changed women and that women have changed medicine, this report includes an appendix expanding on tables presented in the body of the report.

Apple, Rima D., ed. *Women, Health and Medicine in America: A Historical Handbook.* New York: Garland, 1990.
This collection of essays, mentioned in Chapter 2, "Care of Women," is particularly pertinent for this chapter in that it deals with the history of women in the health care professions. Its contributions in the fourth section—"Health Care Providers," "Midwives and History," "Nurses," "Physicians," and "Pharmacists"—are particularly relevant. Beyond these direct considerations of those who have been clearly seen to be

health care providers, the book provides a section titled "Alternative Medical Care," which deals not only with "Women and Sectarian Medicine" but also with female charismatic and religious leaders who have made a difference in the healing professions. These considerations enable the reader to arrive beyond the divisions still assumed between women who are the givers of health care and women who are the receivers. In addition, it prepares the reader to understand the amount of health care given by women who are neither paid members of the health care professions, nor those who are themselves receiving health care at any particular time.

Blackwell, Dr. Elizabeth. *Pioneer Work in Opening the Medical Profession to Women.* New York: Schocken Books, 1977.

This edition is a republication of the letters of Dr. Elizabeth Blackwell, whom some consider to be the first woman physician in the United States. Blackwell was born in 1821. She pressed for the entry of women into the medical profession in an age when numbers of women went without medical care rather than be examined by a male. She attended Geneva Medical College in New York, having been admitted because the male students, thinking her application a joke, replied with a laughing affirmative. Blackwell's story shows the stumbling blocks for women seeking to enter medicine at her time. Barred from residencies and ignored by colleagues, the women had to create their own hospitals and residency programs. The question of histories and firsts can also be asked by the reader. In a time when only 17% of male physicians attended medical college, the woman considered to be the first female physician in the United States is a graduate of the medical college. In fact, Harriet Hunt was in practice at the time. She learned as did most male physicians in her time, by apprenticeship.

Bowman, Marjorie A., and Deborah I. Allen. *Stress and Women Physicians.* New York: Springer-Verlag, 1985.

This book considers the well-being of female physicians along with the stressors they face, stressors similar to yet different from the challenges of women cracking through the barriers of other professions. Women physicians are still clearly a minority in the profession. While the small minority is growing to a more substantial one, and while medicine as an art and science is evolving, women still face stressors peculiar to minorities. Some of the stressors female physicians face are similar to those of other women in the health care professions who constituted 85% of health care workers in 1975 a majority of numbers, yet a minority of power. The authors begin with a brief history of women in medicine, helpful for a context of the present situation. They present a chapter on "Practice Characteristics of Women Physicians," in which they find that women in medicine are more frequently in salaried positions in institutional settings, have lower income, are more frequently in urban areas, spend more time with their patients, and serve more women, minority, and younger patients. They note that male physicians have a lower than average divorce rate, while female physicians have a higher than average one. Chapter 9 deals specifically with "Female Physician Stress." The authors discuss lack of role models, role strain for the female physician, the role of physicians in general, the role of wife and mother, and the role of self. Providing pointers toward solutions to these strains, the authors offer alternatives which may serve to spark the reader's imagination to new options.

Brown, Joanne Carlson, and Carole R. Bohm, eds. *Christianity, Patriarchy, and Abuse*. New York: The Pilgrim Press, 1990.

This second printing, the original being in 1989, questions, in multiple ways, whether Christianity is so tied to patriarchy that, rather than challenging violence and suffering, it glorifies these and makes them holy. A related question is whether, in fact, it is possible to be feminist and still be a participant in the Christian tradition. The contributors to this collection of essays offer healing care for women through their efforts to address these two questions through the lenses of theology, history, ethics, and psychology. They do so by grappling with painful questions, all the more painful for them as these questions strike at the very heart of the Christian tradition. The book falls rather flowingly into three sections, the first dealing with theological questions and historical perspectives, the second considering more specific ethical/theological considerations, and the third providing a view through psychological lenses. While the essays, written by recognized thinkers and researchers, are all interconnected, any one of them can be read with great profit on its own terms. For those employed in the healing professions, perhaps the most helpful, practically speaking, of the essays are Reuther's "The Western Tradition and Violence Against Women," Bloomquist's "Sexual Violence: Patriarchy's Offense and Defense," Redmond's "Christian 'Virtues' and Recovery from Child Sexual Abuse," and Fortune's "The Transformation of Suffering: A Biblical and Theological Perspective". One can derive great profit from reading this book in conjunction with Pamela Cooper-White, *The Cry of Tamar* (Fortress Press, 1995) and Miranda Davies, *Women and Violence* (Zed Books, 1994).

Carlson, Karen J., M.D., Stephanie A. Eisenstadt, M.D., and Terra Ziporyn, Ph.D. *The Harvard Guide to Women's Health.* Cambridge, MA: Harvard University Press, 1996.

While this book fits appropriately into Chapter 5 on "Self-Education and Self-Help," its existence is a prime example of the unity of care of women and care by women. With over 300 entries, written in clear and understandable English, it is the work of women doctors offering companionship to, educating, and supporting women in their health concerns. It deals with care of women's health and reveals education and communicative writing as care by women in the health professions. Combining medical knowledge, critical guidance, and hard to locate data with pioneering information in the field of women's primary care, this book places women's whole health across the lifespan into the hands of the women concerned.

Conn, Joann Wolski, ed. *Women's Spirituality: Resources for Christian Development.* Mahwah, NJ: Paulist Press, 1996.

This second edition of *Women's Spirituality* is a collection of essays demonstrating the integration between spiritual and psychological development from the point of view of women's experience. As health care becomes more aware of the place of spirituality in the healing process, the work of research reflecting upon spiritual experience and making it available to women by women is a particular mode of care. This book is presented in four sections "Issues in Women's Spirituality," "Women's Psychological Development," "Characteristics of Religious Development," and "Revisioning the Tradition of Christian Spirituality." While it is specifically Christian in tone and intent, the book has helpful insights for women of many traditions and no tradition. Its roster of contributors is stunning, and it offers much to spiritual companions, counselors, and therapists as well as women in general.

Cook, Ellen Piel, ed. *Women, Relationships, and Power: Implications for Counseling.* Alexandria, VA: American Counseling Association, 1993.

While this book is directly about counseling and highlight implications of data and dynamics, it considers a number of women's health issues and is pointed toward professionals who care for women. The collection of essays considers issues such as balancing relationships with career, depression, reproduction, eating disorders as well as other addictions, and internalized misogyny. The "Conclusion: Helping Women Heal, Today and Tomorrow" is a fitting close for reminding the reader of the context of the book. It can be helpful to the reader to read any particular essay in tandem with other entries in this bibliography, for example, the essay "Women and Their Bodies: Eating Disorders and Addictions" is profitably read in tandem with Joan Jacobs Brumberg, *Fasting Girls* (Harvard University Press, 1988), "The Impact of Internalized Misogyny and Violence Against Women on Feminine Identity" is well read side by side with Anna Kosof, *Battered Women*

(Franklin Watts, 1994), and with Miranda Davies, *Women and Violence: Realities and Responses Worldwide* (Zed Books, 1995).

Dossey, Barbara. "Healing Partnerships." In *Spirituality and Health Care.* Albuquerque: University of New Mexico Press, 1997.

Basing her discussion on interconnectedness as vital to healing, the author considers "Eras of Medicine," materialistic, mind/body, and nonlocal states of consciousness. Moving from a bio-psycho-social model to a bio-psycho-social-spiritual model, Dossey considers "The Healing System" and "Physiology and the Human Spirit." Dossey ends her considerations with "Creating Healing Rituals." Particularly helpful is her set of self-assessment questions. Speaking in terms of presence and healing, Dossey passes on a wonderful insight concerning the word "partner" from the old English. That consideration sets the context for the whole of her discussion.

Fogel, Catherine Ingram, and Nancy Fugate Woods, eds. *Women's Health Care: A Comprehensive Handbook.* Thousand Oaks, CA: Sage Publications, 1995.

Chapter 2, "Women as Health Care Providers," opens the question of care by women, including considerations upon women as unpaid providers of health care. Connected ideas about, and implications of, the considerations of women as health care providers are contained in Chapter 7, "Women and Health Care," and, Chapter 8, "Frameworks for Nursing Practice with Women." While these chapters speak most directly about care by women, all contributing essays reflect, in some way, the implications of the data and insights concerned, as these pertain to health care providers, most particularly nurses.

Goodrich, Thelma Jean, ed. *Women and Power: Perspectives for Family Therapy.* New York: W. W. Norton and Company, 1991.

This analysis, which recognizes power as a central organizing principle in families, explores ways of addressing women's usually disadvantaged position with regard to this reality. In addition to Goodrich's powerful opening chapter, Part I contains an essay by Jean Baker Miller, "Women and Power: Reflections Ten years Later." Particularly pertinent are Part III, "Story and Ritual," which considers the manner in which women get and develop personal authority through self-stories and ritual, and Part IV, "Family Therapy," which presents a chapter on "Power Politics in Therapy with Women" by Judith Myers Avis. This work, at the same time that it challenges definitions of power, demands empowerment for women. While it pursues that demand, it does not lose sight of the day-to-day struggles which both the client and the therapist must engage.

Gornick, Lisa. "Developing a New Narrative: The Woman Therapist and the Male Patient." In *Psychoanalysis and Women: Contemporary Reappraisals.* Hillsdale, NJ: The Analytic Press, 1986.
Gathering data from in-depth interviews with female therapists about their work with male patients, Gornick shows that the different meanings of power and sexuality for men and for women are critical for understanding the interaction in the client/therapist dyad. Gornick claims that when a woman is the therapist she steps out of the feminine role, this reversal of power having implications for transference. The woman's authority may be a sign that she may not be approached sexually. Her authority may be experienced as either threatening or belittling to the patient's masculinity. Gornick then discusses countertransference issues for the female therapist. She may feel threatened or guilty in response to the erotic transference. She may feel frustrated at being cast as the bad mother. Gornick's insight sheds light, especially in terms of the balance of power she is addressing, on transference and countertransference issues. It also points toward the societal attitudes which make these issues a question.

Hamilton, Alice. *Exploring the Dangerous Trades.* Boston: Little Brown and Company, 1943.
This autobiographical work, among other things, tells the story of the

physician who was *par excellence*, the expert on industrial diseases in her time. Part of her story gives the current reader a glimpse of history as well as a personal experience with which she or he may not be familiar. Hamilton was selected as assistant professor at Harvard's School of Medicine in a time when no woman could be accepted into that program. Situated in a branch of medicine which had gained in importance because of the Second World War, but had not attracted men, Hamilton was clear that she was chosen because she was really the only candidate available. She was clearly instructed that her appointment was not to be considered as any precedent for admitting women to Harvard's Medical School, nor were the trustees about to reconsider the question of coeducation at that school. Hamilton was apprised of three limitations upon her faculty membership. She was not allowed in the faculty club, she was not to participate in academic processions at commencement, and she was not eligible for faculty tickets to football games. One of the results of her status at Harvard was that fifteen years after her arrival there, she became the only *assistant* professor emeritus in the history of the school. Reading this book in conjunction with Abram, *"Send Us a Lady Physician": Women Doctors in America, 1835-1920* (W. W. Norton and Company, 1985), and Karen J. Carlson et al., *The Harvard Guide to Women's Health* (Harvard University Press, 1996), provides an interesting historical journey.

Hine, Darlene Clark. "Co-Laborers in the Work of the Lord: Nineteenth-Century Black Women Physicians." In Ruth J. Abram, ed., *"Send Us a Lady Physician": Women Doctors in America, 1835-1920*. New York: W. W. Norton and Company, 1985.
    Pointing to the fact that there are only scattered bits and pieces of information regarding Afro-American women physicians of the late nineteenth and early twentieth centuries, Hines is able to say that in the twenty-five years after the end of slavery, there were 115 black female physicians in the United States. She points to the Afro-American women graduates of the Women's Medical College of Pennsylvania and of the

post-Reconstruction black medical schools in the South of the United States: Howard, Meharry, Leonard, and Flint. She provides the stories of Dr. Caroline Still Wiley Anderson, Dr. Eliza Grier, Dr. Halle Tanner Dillon Johnson, and Dr. Mathilde Evans, among others. Black women physicians were an integral part of the communities in which they practiced, founding a number of health care institutions.

Hurd-Mead, Kate Campbell. *A History of Women in Medicine, from the Earliest Times to the Beginning of the Nineteenth Century.* Haddam, CT: Haddam Press, 1938.

Hurd-Mead, encouraged by Sir William Osler to seek out the place of women in the development of medicine, found the information meager. Such a study had not been undertaken previously, and any information available was in medical histories written by men. Busy with her private practice, the author collected information between 1890 and 1925. At that time, she relinquished her practice; researched, at the British Museum library, early documents in their original languages; and compiled as true and complete a story as she could. She then examined manuscripts in other libraries; made personal visits to most of the countries of Europe, Africa, and Asia; and kept up correspondence over a period of years with women physicians. This book is the result of that research. Hurd-Mead presents a detailed and chronological history.

Learn, Cheryl Demerath. *Older Women's Experience of Spirituality: Crafting the Quilt.* New York: Garland, 1996.

In this work, Learn attends to the spirituality of older women, the fastest growing part of the American population. In a phenomenological study, she investigates the experience of spirituality and spiritual caring of eight women over the age of seventy. In reflecting upon the transcribed data, Learn finds five essential emerging features: choosing solitude, connecting with community, dialoging with presence, re-creating the self, and encountering spiritual caring. Using the metaphor of a quilt and actually reinforcing the metaphor by the crafting of a quilt, the author makes a significant contribution to nursing research, theory, practice, and education. In making her considerations upon methodology Learn mentions her researcher's perspective making explicit three areas which bear upon her inquiry: institutional church and spirituality, women older than herself, and feminism and feminist theology. In these experiences and concerns, the author shares much with most of her readers.

Leeson, Joyce, and Judith Gray. *Women and Medicine*. London: Tavistock, 1978.

This book concerns not only woman doctors but all women health care workers in addition, as well as those who receive health care services. It examines the relationships between the sexes in the health care industry, noting that doctors are predominantly male, mostly middle-class members of a respected profession. Patients tend to be working class and non-professionals. Women patients, differing also by gender, experience yet one more dimension of social distance between themselves and the male doctor. The authors note that women physicians are subject to a number of contradictory pressures, by virtue of being both physician and female. Ultimately, Leeson and Gray find three major barriers between doctors and other health care providers, and doctors and patients. These are between class, profession, and sex. They find that the least explored barrier is that of sex. As early as the publication time of this book, researchers such as Leeson and Gray were well aware that the health care industry is primarily staffed by women workers. In an industry so work intensive and so inserted into the low paid sector, these women have held, by and large, subservient and supportive roles. While this phenomenon is not isolated and holds true generally in society, it sometimes appears less obvious in the health care sector. This book is divided into three parts: "Women Providers of Health Care," "Women Users of Health Services," and "Women Get Organized."

Levin, Beatrice. *Women and Medicine: Pioneers Meeting the Challenge*. Lincoln, NE: Media Publishing, 1988.

Containing a history of United States and Canadian women physicians, this book reveals that history by telling the stories of a number of women physicians. It does so with a warmth and whimsy, as well as an eye to the international. It is in the telling of the stories that women's health issues and human status are mentioned. In this work, women's health is woven into a history of women physicians in modern times. While Levin recounts issues of discrimination, women's brilliant medical careers and Nobel prizes, and changing cultural attitudes, her writing is a reminder that equal opportunity for women in the field, recent concept that it is, is still in a fragile position. Her treatment of the combined roles of women in the medical profession and her multicultural approach leave room for many women to see themselves as in a mirror. Her historical perspectives on Jewish, Arab, and Greek women in medicine provide data not easily located by the ordinary reader, yet contextualized by a chatty making of the connections. Housed in Part V; "Promises to Keep," Levin's Chapter 25, "Health Care in the Land of the Free," provides a helpful entree into the questions of health care reform in the United States.

Lewis, Judith A., and Judith Bernstein. *Women's Health: A Relational Perspective Across the Life Cycle.* Boston: Jones and Bartlett, 1996.
This work, written for nursing or women's studies, is a response to a felt need for its perspective. Noting excellent books addressing women's health from a medical perspective, as well as excellent books addressing women's growth and development, the authors filled a need by wedding these two perspectives in one volume. It is an interdisciplinary historical, sociocultural, biophysiological and psychosocial approach offering a women-centered view. Part I sets the context by providing a theoretical and historical framework, appreciating the strengths of women and exploring gender, class, and race with regard to health. Part II, considering women's maturation from a life cycle perspective, addresses adolescence, the reproductive years, perimenopause, and aging. Its emphasis is on maintaining health and wellness. Part III discusses the

complexity of women's roles. It offers the reader a global context and includes case studies of women's situations in Panama and South Africa. This section ends with Chapter 13, "Developing a New Model for the Care of Women." The ten tenets for a new covenant between women and their health care providers (pp. 331-332) is not only a challenge but also an excellent way of stating the continuing direction which the authors see as necessary to the furtherance of women's health care.

Lopate, Carol. *Women in Medicine.* Baltimore, MD: The Johns Hopkins University Press, 1968.

In this book, summarizing the experience of being a woman physician in the United States, Lopate makes suggestions for improvements in women's situation in the medical field. She makes the case for changing the national climate with regard to sexual roles, so that both genders can attain their full personal potential. Published in 1968, the work cannot allude to the changes of the most recent history of female physicians. That very fact is helpful to the reader in that the book provides a look at the status and concerns, the obstacles, and the cultural climate vis-à-vis women at the end of the 1960s. This book was a result of the Macy Conference convened in 1966. Educators and physicians came together then to discuss the underutilization of woman power in the United States as that underutilization pertained to the medical shortage at that time. Surprised at how little pertinent information was available, the group suggested an independent study, this book. The work, intended for women considering medical careers, their advisors, and their teachers, facilitates more informed career decisions as well as an understanding of the problems and possibilities for professional women.

Lorber, Judith. *Women Physicians: Career, Status, and Power.* New York: Tavistock, 1984.

The Association of American Medical Colleges did a twenty-year longitudinal study of the class of 1960. This book combines that survey with personal interviews of physicians affiliated with a metropolitan medical center's department of internal medicine. The work traces the development of careers of contemporary women physicians in the United States. The author points out the consequences of continued discrimination vis-à-vis the possibilities of women physicians' competing for top positions. She suggests strategies for overcoming the situation. There is also consideration of the effects of family and children on women and their careers. Particularly helpful is a comparison with women physicians in England and in the Soviet Union. The comparison shows similarities in career patterns. The two appendices of the book document the personal interviews and the results of the AAMC survey.

McClain, Carol Shepherd, ed. *Women as Healers: Cross-Cultural Perspectives*. New Brunswick, NJ: Rutgers University Press, 1989.
Opening with "Reinterpreting Women in Healing Roles," this work is presented in four parts: "Women as Informal Healers," "Healing with Female Metaphors," "Women as Ritual Specialists," and "Women Healers and Culture Change." Its integrated approach discusses women in Andean communities, in Sri Lanka, in Korea, in Puerto Rico, in Southern Africa, and in the United States. Its contributors approach issues as diverse as family healing, shamanism, and midwifery. This book considers the differences between medical anthropology and the anthropology of women. It is at once scholarly and experiential, sophisticated and clear. Its representation of women's healing across cultural, geographical, economic, and social boundaries makes clear the diversity and connectedness of women.

Melosh, Barbara. "Every Woman Is a Nurse: Work and Gender in the Emergence of Nursing." In Ruth J. Abram, ed., *"Send Us a Lady Physician": Women Doctors in America, 1835-1920*. New York: W. W. Norton and Company, 1985.
The title of this essay is taken from Florence Nightingale's *Notes on Nursing*, which was pointed toward women in families. The author makes the case that even in the technological situation of contemporary

hospitals and nursing, the cultural ideology of "woman's solace" still colors the division of labor for health care. She then gives a brief and clear history of modern professional nursing. This story includes the founding of nursing schools, the growth of hospitals, the changing market, and the helps and hazards of professionalization. Melosh makes some interesting comparisons between the situation of the female doctor and the situation of the nurse. Her observations on the erosion of the autonomy of the medical profession are interesting and raise pertinent questions for women in the health care professions. This essay is well read in conjunction with Barbara Ehrenreich and Deirdre English, *Witches, Midwives, and Nurses*, Feminist Press, 1973.

Melosh, Barbara. *"The Physician's Hand": Work Culture and Conflict in American Nursing*. Philadelphia: Temple University Press, 1982.
The work culture, that is, the rules, lore, and behavior connected to a distinct work or work site, is the set of lenses through which Melosh presents this history of nursing from the 1920s to the 1970s. The author concentrates on women's experience rather than on a distanced analysis of the field of nursing. She includes chapters discussing the outcomes of professionalization, the history and culture of hospital schools and other institutions, public health nursing, and private duty nursing. In considering the impact which feminism has exercised with regard to changes in nursing, the author looks to future questions as nurses assume more responsibility and are identified as patient advocates.

Morantz-Sanchez, Regina Markell. *Sympathy and Science: Women Physicians in American Medicine*. New York: Oxford University Press, 1985.
Through the use of excerpts from diaries and from letters, Morantz-Sanchez concretizes a history of women medical practitioners from colonial to contemporary times. She shows nineteenth century women moving into the public arena and describes their formal medical

education as one part of that move. The work considers female physicians' involvement in reform movements, their dealing with conflicts between family demands and professional ones, their drop in numbers after 1910, their low visibility from the 1930s to the 1960s, and their growth in numbers confluent with feminism of the 1960s on. The author's research on women and the development of obstetrics is interesting. She does not conclude, as some have, that early female physicians were opposed to gynecological surgery while male surgeons endorsed it. She does, however, show obstetrics, pediatrics, and public health as feminine medical specialties of the late nineteenth century. She points to women's excellence in background and skills for obstetrics resulting from their training in female medical colleges and women-run hospitals, and she points to women physicians' work with women and children as being seen as improving the moral fiber of society.

Neuger, Christie Cozad, ed. *The Arts of Ministry: Feminist-Womanist Approaches.* Louisville, KY: Westminster John Knox Press, 1996.
Intended to speak to the actual practice of ministry from feminist and womanist perspectives, this book encourages apprenticeship models while at the same time admitting that most apprenticeship opportunities have not yet developed practice congruent with feminist and womanist thought. This collection of essays invites this as yet undeveloped practice by attending to the art of ministry in a way somewhat analogous to that in which medical practitioners have been attending to the art of medicine. The contributors engrave their invitation by considering pastoral care, preaching, education, pastoral counseling, administration, ethics, and mentoring. The writing is characterized by clarity and readability. It can be readily understood by professionals and non-professionals alike, an excellent practical quality born of thirty years of thought and struggle in the community of ministerial women.

Northrup, Christiane, M.D. "Menopause." In *Women's Bodies, Women's Wisdom.* New York: Bantam Books, 1995.

Northrup begins her discussion of menopause with considerations upon our cultural inheritance. She deals with hormones, fear of aging, types of menopause, and symptoms of menopause. Her approach is one eminently respectful to the reader, providing information and experience but leaving decisions to the reader. Weaving spirituality and sensible sifting through her presentation, she maintains a holistic approach. Northrup presents considerations on natural menopause and phytoestrogens, natural hormones in food as well as artificial menopause and synthetic estrogen replacement therapy. Particularly helpful to some readers are the pages on osteoporosis. The presentation is clear and the information direct. The author looks at screening methods for bone density, as well as nutritional and exercise approaches for bone health. In her treatment of mood swings and depression, she considers the experience of "fuzzy thinking." She also provides a discussion on ERT (estrogen replacement therapy), on breast cancer, and on heart disease all particularly pertinent to menopause. Perhaps most practically helpful to the reader is her listing under "Self Care During Menopause."

Northrup, Christiane, M.D. *Women's Bodies, Women's Wisdom: Creating Physical and Emotional Health and Healing.* New York: Bantam Books, 1995.

This insightful and practical book is an integration of pertinent data, a reemergence of the feminine in healing, a restoration of spirituality to medicine, and a presentation of holistic knowledge across broad areas. Its clarity and readability as well as its tables, illustrations, and listings of resources make it convenient as a sourcebook. The author's rediscovery, recognition, and use of wisdom with science is an approach that resounds with many women. The book, based on the dynamics of Women to Women, founded by the author, another ob/gyn, and two nurse practitioners, encourages listening to and trusting one's body. It presents stories of healing told in women's words and images. It encourages women to "name" and "reclaim" their lives by finding voice and giving voice. Chapter 15, "Steps for Healing," for example, presents wisdom and encourages voice such that it can be used in relationship to any unhealed place, physical, spiritual, or biopsychosocial.

Slayton, Tamara. *Reclaiming the Menstrual Matrix: Evolving Feminine Wisdom–A Workbook.* Petaluma, CA: Menstrual Health Foundation, 1990. Slayton discusses what has been, and is still, for many women a negative experience - menopause. Her positive presentation of the climacteric as a surge of energy and an expression of the power and wisdom available at a special time for women invites the discovery of a new and vital identity rather than the negative results of energy turned inward upon oneself. She sees the need for women to confront the culture's lack of information and misinformation concerning this life event, and she encourages women to address nutritional needs unique to menopause and to move into a deeper, freer self-experience. Slayton addresses the wisdom years after menopause, interweaving into her considerations information on myths and rites of passage from different cultures. She considers the unique gifts brought to the community by women in their postmenopausal years. She encourages a rediscovery of the true meaning of menopause hidden behind the reversals and degradations of its meaning which still hold sway.

Smith, Susan L. *Sick and Tired of Being Sick and Tired: Black Women's Health Activism in America, 1890-1950.* Philadelphia: University of Pennsylvania Press, 1995.
Begun in 1985 as a seminar paper and having grown into a master's thesis in 1986 and a doctoral dissertation in 1991, this book addresses Black women's health activism in a variety of ways. Its introduction provides an excellent historical context, an eye-opener for most readers. Pointing to the unbroken and continuous line of this activism since the 1890s, the author shows Black female professionals, as well as community leaders, founding health projects and implementing health reform measures at the local level. She is clear about Black women's

influence on the health of their families and is forthright about Black laywomen's key role and ongoing contributions. One of the beauties of this book is that it is "the first full-scale effort to examine health reform initiatives created by African Americans themselves" (p. 12). In the first section, "The Creation of a Black Health Movement," Smith traces the development of a black health movement of the twentieth century. The second section, "The Implementation of Black Health Programs," follows with an exploration of health reform in Alabama and Mississippi. The author concludes with noticing ways in which Black women's community organizing for health continued after 1950, wrapping her conclusions in the words of Fannie Lou Hamer about Black people being "sick and tired of being sick and tired." Surely this phrase fits any number of women dealing with health care for their loved ones.

Snow, Loudell F. *Walkin' Over Medicine*. San Francisco: Westview Press, 1993.
Written by a professor of anthropology and adjunct professor of pediatrics and human development, this book treats the combination of folk medicine and biomedicine used in African American communities. Studying African American health beliefs and practices over the greater part of professional life, this author understands the extraordinary people who have dealt on a daily basis with the ailments of body, mind, and spirit of those who have approached them for help. This complementary combination of traditional faith healing, herbal medicine, and medical establishment drugs has served communities well. The author researches and understands with a sympathy leading to wisdom, and with an appreciation leading to admiration. The anthropologist's eye sees the purposes and effects of traditional healing, and the pediatrics and human development teacher's eye sees the purposes and effect of establishment medicine. In both cases, Snow sees clearly the healing effects of folk medicine, even when cure is not possible, and appreciates the empowerment involved.

Solari-Twadell, Phyllis, Anne Marie Djupe, and Mary Ann McDermott, eds. *Parish Nursing: The Developing Practice*. Park Ridge, IL: Lutheran General Health Care System, 1990.

Representing the work of those who have been pioneers in developing parish nursing, this book identifies the context for its developing practice. It considers the models and emerging settings of practice, as well as relevant issues and concerns. The book is written to be read not only by nursing and clergy professionals but by congregations and congregational leaders, such as finance committee members. This becomes clear in the first section, which deals with context, and comprises essays titled "The Mission of Health and the Congregation," "A Historical Perspective: Holistic Health and the Parish Nurse," and "Society, the Parish and the Parish Nurse." Aimed at developing collaborative practice, the book provides essays on "Team Ministry in the Parish" and on "Pastoral Reflections." The emphasis on the congregation as a locus of care points out the importance of the community in healing.

Strehlow, Wighard, and Gottfried Hertzka. *Hildegard of Bingen's Medicine*. Santa Fe, NM: Bear and Company, 1988.

The German authors of this book, a medical doctor and a research chemist, extract from Hildegard's works her medical knowledge. Experimenting with her remedies on a large scale, they found them to be effective. The book is a reference work, intended as a source of general information, integrating Hildegard's natural herbal medicine with spiritual knowledge. The book provides a renewed understanding of the roots of Western herbal medicine and natural-healing tradition. It also provides a spiritual focus for healing apt for bringing many back to cultural origins. The book, in fifteen chapters, also provides appendices and indices which are very helpful in offering background to the reader.

Thomas, Zach. *Healing Touch: The Church's Forgotten Language*. Louisville, KY: Westminster John Knox Press, 1994.

While this book does not consider care by women directly, its call for the rediscovery of touch in healing ministries points toward a return to holism in ministerial perspectives. This has been a concern of women in the healing professions: nurses, spiritual companions, counselors, massage therapists, and physicians. The author of this work refers to touch as a healing force and as a mode of sharing compassion: in informal relationships; in formal professional settings, including those of bodyworkers and therapists; and in worship. Part 1 deals with "Touch in Western Healing Traditions." Part 2 considers "Touch in Modern Ministry." In its Appendix A, this book provides "Reflection Sheets." It also provides a "Bibliography" and "Resources." Thomas Zach's interest in healing of the whole person is congruent with approaches to health care by women.

Wallace, Ruth A. *They Call Her Pastor: A New Role for Catholic Women.* Albany: State University of New York Press, 1992.

This book presents a sociological study of "priestless" Catholic parishes headed by women in the United States. The description of female pastors at these parishes focuses on collaborative leadership practices by women, their unique qualities as pastors, gender inequality in the church, and the constraints and support systems related to these women. The author presents her information in a clear and moving manner, having seen at first hand the work of these pastors. She traveled to their parishes, accompanied them on their pastoral visitations, and took part in the community gatherings around such occasions as baptisms, weddings, and parish dinners. Wallace's Chapter 9, "Final Observations," dreams beyond the trailblazing phenomenon of these women, while at the same time acknowledging and respecting their contributions.

Walsh, Mary Roth. *"Doctors Wanted: No Women Need Apply": Sexual Barriers in the Medical Profession, 1835-1975.* New Haven, CT: Yale University Press, 1977.

Walsh's delving into women's past in the medical profession showed her that nineteenth century female physicians in the United States were, far from being an anomaly, a remarkably growing number by the end of that century. Her research showed her the cultural roots of sexism with regard to this question. Rather than fade away, the institutional barriers of sexism stayed resilient in the twentieth century, turning back the tide of women who aspired to careers in medicine. Showing that the medical establishment made conscious efforts to minimize the number of women physicians, Walsh points to its success in the statistical drop in those numbers between 1890 and 1950. This book not only explores why women have not been given an equal chance in medicine, it also stands as a warning that hard-won victories for professional women are easily wiped away. Chapter 8, "What Went Wrong," and Chapter 9, "Will History Repeat Itself?," tend to these latter two insights. Since only women pursuing regular medicine are documented in Walsh's book, the reader might want to consider it in tandem with Ruth J. Abram, *"Send Us a Lady Physician": Women Doctors in America* (W. W. Norton and Company, 1985) to get a sense of those involved in irregular medicine.

Westberg, Granger, with Jill Westberg McNamara. *The Parish Nurse.* Park Ridge, IL: Parish Nurse Resource Center, 1987.
This book offers a creative way for congregations to provide a holistic ministry to their members. It encourages a program bringing nurses onto parish staffs to work as ministers of health care. Explaining the what and the why of a parish nursing program, Westberg shows the parish nurse as a bridge between science and religion. He provides practical resources such as a whole person health inventory, sample job descriptions, models and types of parish nurse services, and a rural parish church network. Westberg shows how congregations can play an important role in keeping members spiritually and physically healthy, at the same time that he provides leadership in the field of preventive medicine.

White, Evelyn C., ed. *The Black Women's Health Book: Speaking for Ourselves.* Seattle: Seal Press, 1994.
This expanded edition of the original 1990 publication is a continuing response to connection and to health among black women. It contains an update on HIV infection and black women, as well as an essay on Nurse Rivers. With new additions on fibroids, breast feeding, non-Western medicine, menopause, the evolution of the African American diet, and the challenges black women face within medical settings, this work features the writing of more than fifty black women on the health issues affecting them, their families, and their communities. The information and writing are powerful and the range of issues is expansive.

Winter, Miriam Therese. *WomanWord: A Feminist Lectionary and Psalter, Women of the New Testament.* New York: Crossroad, 1990.
Recognizing the meaning-making power of ritual, this book also recognizes that history, written by the winners, ordinarily leaves out the losers. In rituals molded only by male perceptions and interpretations, images and symbols reflect and reinforce gender inequality. Winter considers that real gender mutuality cannot happen until fundamental assumptions at the heart of present patriarchal religious ritual change at the root. She offers the reader rituals which touch upon the inner truth of women and help in their quest for integration. She supplies women with other women's stories, reminding us of those women who have gone before. The diversity of appeal to women's experience in this work can be seen in some of the titles of the psalms: "A Psalm on Behalf of the Poor," "A Psalm of Bringing to Birth," "A Mother-in-Law's Psalm," "A Psalm for Women Who Are Abused," "A Psalm for Women in Leadership," and "A Little Girl's Psalm." This work is beautifully illustrated by Meinrad Craighead.

Yount, Lisa. *Contemporary Women Scientists*. New York: Facts on File, 1994.

Have women in science come a long way in this century? Partially, yes. The ten women included in this book are indicative of the increase of women in medical studies, in the physical sciences, and in mathematics. While the more obvious problems of the past seem to have dissolved, the current problems for women scientists are now more subtle, and thus, more difficult to address. Women in the scientific fields name the "glass ceiling," "old boys clubs," and "science nuns," a term for the belief that a woman cannot handle a family and a demanding career, as beliefs and practices still afoot. Of particular interest for this bibliography are four of the scientists. Helen Brooke Taussig, a pediatric cardiologist at Johns Hopkins in the 1940s, invented an operation which saved the lives of babies born with heart defects. Gertrude Bell Elion, a chemist, in 1951 developed the first drug to fight cancer successfully by interfering with the nucleic acid of those cells. Jewel Plummer Cobb, successful in cancer research, teaching, and college administration, contributed to science's understanding of melanoma. Candace Beebe Pert, a neuroscientist who made breakthrough studies of brain chemicals and their receptors, has gleaned important information on how mind and body may communicate.

SELF-EDUCATION AND SELF-HELP

INTRODUCTION

It becomes difficult to devise a chapter which is exclusively devoted to self-education and self-help with regard to women and health, since a large part of the progress in this enterprise has come from the "bottom up." That is, women demanding that something about the distancing of the "experts" be removed and that they know well and care for their bodies, was, in fact, the major breakthrough both in women's studies in general and in women's health in particular. In terms of education, women, in some way, wrested health knowledge from the halls of the hospitals and the halls of ivy. Sometimes grass roots women's knowledge was not so different from that of the professionals, but their approach was neither to accept nor to use obfuscating jargon in speaking of women's health. In doing so, they midwived new epistemologies which chose not to confuse lack of intelligibility with heightened sophistication.

A corresponding dynamic in self-education and self-help came from the recovery movement in general and women's needs vis-à-vis recovery in particular. Thus, a number of early self-education and self-help works can be credited to addictions recovery. Again, that movement came from the "bottom up," from the very people who found themselves suffering from addiction (originally, alcoholism). Those individuals and groups found workable health approaches and explained them to researchers, and eventually this information arrived in the medical and other health professions. While there is a parallel dynamic at work in women's self-help books and addictions self-help books, the addictions books are placed in a separate section.

While the books in "Care of Women" and "Care by Women" in this annotated bibliography can clearly be useful for women's self-education and our use toward self-help, the books in this chapter tend not to address specialists or publicly recognized professionals, although they can also be helpful to that community. The books in this chapter tend to be more overt and more direct concerning the mind/body connection in language accessible to all readers. Ultimately, because of the integrative aspects of women's health, as well as the integrative aspects of how the knowledge has been acquired, "Care of Women," "Care by Women," and "Self-Education and Self-Help" can also be read as one. The aspects explained above also account for the relative brevity of this chapter.

ANNOTATIONS

Aisenberg, Nadyna, and Mona Harrington. *Women of Academe: Outsiders in the Sacred Grove*. Amherst: University of Massachusetts Press, 1988.
This book recommends that women in academe learn about the status of women in that profession, seek the support of other women colleagues, and plan strategically for their careers. One beauty of this study is that its authors are independent scholars looking at why so few women succeed, that is, gain tenure at major academic institutions. Aisenberg and Harrington's study is built upon interviews with sixty women academics who share their experiences, which the authors conclude show professional marginalization and exclusion from the centers of power in academe. An appendix, providing background information on the interviewees follows the authors' "Epilogue: Four Lives," personal accounts by the four women academics mentioned in that section. While this work does not deal directly with women's self-education and self-help with regard to health issues, it provides experiences and strategies transferrable from educational systems to health systems, history and ideas concerning women's education, and strategic thought toward help and support in any profession in which women find themselves.

Beattie, Melody. *Codependent No More*. Center City, MN: Hazelden, 1987.

In the style of self-help books, this one gives not only pertinent information but also pragmatic conclusions with respect to responses to addictive behaviors. In a sense, the book is a double-edged sword. It provides help in naming and coping with problems arising from relationships with addicted persons. It also names as personally problematic, if not almost pathological, behaviors which have not only been culturally attributed to but also mightily encouraged in women. Beattie also does well in walking the tightrope between liberating information and unwittingly inviting encouragement toward "blaming the victim." In any event, women are well served by this book both by its insightful information and by its pragmatic empowerment.

Bermosk, Loretta S., and Sarah E. Porter. *Women's Health and Human Wholeness*. New York: Appleton-Century-Crofts, 1979.

Among some of the earlier approaches to holistic health concepts and multicultural approaches, this book is easily readable and provides a focus for women's self-reflection upon their own experiences of body.

Borysenko, Joan, Ph.D. *Minding the Body, Mending the Mind*. New York: Bantam Books, 1988.

Approaching her work from the perspective of mind/body oneness, Borysenko provides a delightful amount of information and opportunity for the reader to exercise the learnings of the book. A pioneer in psychoneuroimmunology and co-founder of the Mind/Body Clinic with Dr. Ilan Kutz, Dr. Borysenko, in a short time, became director. Her work has pursued the integration of traditional treatments with contemporary alternatives. It is just such discoveries which the author presents. Beginning with a chapter on "The Science of Healing," Borysenko encourages the reader to reclaim and reframe so that relaxation, serenity, and in-chargeness can return to the self. Most helpful in terms of the continuing tools for self-education and self-help are Chapter 6,

"Reframing and Creative Imagination," and Chapter 7, "Healing the Emotions." "Suggestions for the Reader" at the end of each chapter are practical and pointed. Her "Epilogue," containing twelve brief reminders, is a wonderful review of the book's learnings and is enhanced by the "Self-Assessment" which follows. Borysenko provides a list for further reading, supplying a varied selection respectful of the diversity of her readers.

Boston Women's Health Book Collective. *The New Our Bodies, Ourselves*. New York: Touchstone, 1993.

An old favorite that remains an essential resource for women wanting to take control of their bodies and their health. The first *Our Bodies, Ourselves* was published in 1969, with a new edition in 1973. The revision of the second edition in 1976 saw a number of reaches into other nations, saw Spanish speaking women working on translations, and saw the book translated into seven volumes of Braille. The experience of the collaborators was that very shortly after the publication of a new edition, its material might no longer be up-to-date. *The New Our Bodies, Ourselves*, published in 1984, includes earlier prefaces which are enlightening in terms of the history of this work, and the visions and reasons behind it. Particularly enlightening is Preface I, "A Good Story," written originally in March, 1973. This edition contains entirely new chapters on body image, alcohol and other drugs, alternative health care options, psychotherapy, environmental and occupational health, violence against women, new reproductive technologies, women growing older, and international awareness. There are truths, attitudes, and approaches in each of the editions which are never out of date and still give a power, a learning, and a context for updated data. In each of the editions, the discovery of women's power in their own health and their aptitude for researching, claiming, and making their own decisions are paramount. In each, the resources for reading, the networking information and the illustrations, tables, and data are superb. A particularly helpful set of data as well as a contextualizing influence is "The Politics of Women and Medical Care" in the 1984 edition.

Carlson, Karen J., M.D., Stephanie A. Eisenstadt, M.D., and Terra Ziporyn, Ph.D. *The Harvard Guide to Women's Health.* Cambridge, MA: Harvard University Press, 1996.
Besides its clear language, easily navigated alphabetical listings, balanced perspectives, and treatment of overlooked emotional and social issues connected with women's health, this book offers more than 250 illustrations and 400 resources for further information. It provides practical information on description of symptoms and on posing of pointed questions about varying treatment options. Encouraging further study, integration of information, and completeness of understanding, this book supplies a list of related entries after each topic. Its clear and readable style and format encourage perusal. Helpful tables, charts, and diagrams both clarify and review the information presented in prose. The end of each entry lists related topics so that the reader can hone the integrating function of self-education with a natural sense of ease.

Clinebell, Howard, Ph.D. *Well Being: A Personal Plan for Exploring and Enriching the Seven Dimensions of Life.* San Francisco: Harper, 1992.
Naming the seven dimensions of life as mind, body, spirit, love, work, play, and earth, Clinebell presents a series of data, reflections, strategies, and encouragements for the reader. He prefaces his work with "How to Get the Most from this User-Friendly Guide," hoping ultimately to increase in his readers what he calls an "Aliveness Quotient." The book is divided into manageable segments, with periodic "Windows of Wholeness," individuals' stories and insights, delightful cartoons, exercises, checklists, and reminders. Part I of this work involves "Practical Methods for Enhancing Well Being in the Seven Dimensions of Your Life," while Part II deals with "Coping Constructively with Detours, Challenges, and Opportunities on the Journey of Well Being." Clinebell has a unique way of weaving together the work of theologians

and philosophers, health care professionals, therapeutic professionals, and spiritual adepts. The interweaving of these has produced a book deceptively simple by being well-grounded.

Committee on Women's Studies in Asia, eds. *Life Stories of Asian Pioneers in Women's Studies.* New York: The Feminist Press, 1995.
With a foreword by Florence Howe, co-publisher with Kali, this book is an outcome of the Fourth Interdisciplinary Congress on Research on Women at Hunter College. Women of many cultures and situations can recognize themselves in the thirteen memoirs presented in this book. Not only can pioneers recognize the pioneering spirit and accomplishments of one another, but in doing so they can evoke undreamed of changes. Those women whose stories appear in this work have kept the connection between themselves and the least privileged of the women in their countries. This multidisciplinary group of academic women situated at institutes and universities throughout Asia display courage, both personal and political as well as intellectual. The contributors to this volume interweave and integrate women's studies with ongoing social policies of Asian development and committed Third World feminist practice. At the same time that the stories challenge the mind, they touch the heart, so that the reader is invited to find her own courage and action.

Cutler, Winnifred, Ph.D., and Celso-Ramon Garcia, M.D. *Menopause: A Guide for Women and the Men Who Love Them.* Revised edition. New York: W. W. Norton and Company, 1992.
This work includes a "Preface for Men," one filled with biological information as well as sensible approaches to women's experiences of menopause, the chief and first approach being to listen. It points out the prolonged extension of life which has changed medicine and made the considerations around menopause necessary and helpful. The authors encourage the development of a health maintenance plan according to the decisions of the person involved. They reflect upon the changing training process for physicians, pointing out the need for further change.

Proposing self-advocacy and personal responsibility on the part of the patient, the authors discuss the benefits, risks, and side effects of a diversity of treatment and health decision possibilities. This revised edition presents five new chapters on health issues related to menopause: cardiovascular concerns, nutrition, smoking and obesity, exercise, and alternatives to hormone replacement therapy. Practical aids for the reader are presented in a glossary, annual health charts, a bibliography, and clear diagrams and illustrations.

Doress, Paula Brown, Diana Laskin Siegal, and The Midlife and Older Women Book Project, in cooperation with The Boston Women's Health Book Collective. *Ourselves, Growing Older: Women Aging with Knowledge and Power.* New York: Simon and Schuster, 1987. This book is divided into three sections: "Aging Well," "Living with Ourselves and Others as We Age," and "Understanding, Preventing, and Managing Medical Problems." Like its predecessor, *Our Bodies, Ourselves,* it is not only a collaborative effort but also plays an advocacy role. Encouraging self-acceptance, self-worth, creativity, and confidence, this book increases women's ability to stay well, expanding concepts of sisterhood across generations. It encourages the knowledge and sense of taking control of aspects of health which can help older women as well as younger to retain greater independence and responsibility vis-à-vis a health care system which can be confining and sometimes impossible to work with. This health and living handbook takes a proactive and empowering approach to both the physical and emotional health of midlife and older women, presenting frank information. It addresses the potential of the second half of life and includes chapters such as "Aging and Well-Being," "Reassessing Our Body Image," "Contraception and Childbearing at Midlife," "Sexuality in the Middle and Later Years," "Menopause: Entering Our Third Age," "Problems in the Medical Care System," "Osteoporosis, Arthritis, Cancer," "Housing Alternatives and Living Arrangements," "Work and Retirement," and "Money Matters."

As does its predecessor, the book contains excellent tables, illustrations, and resources.

English, Jane Butterfield. *Different Doorway: Adventures of a Caesarian Born.* Point Reyes Station, CA: Earth Heart, 1985.
Butterfield, a physicist, artist, and translator, addresses in transpersonal approaches her experience of birth through non-labor caesarian section. She shares her ten-year journey toward understanding herself through this experience. During that ten years, via dreams, meditation, art, and human potential exercises, Butterfield contextualized this experience, discovering in the process that a birth occurring without labor leaves a specific psychic-spiritual imprint. As planned caesarian sections became more ordinary, the author felt it was time to address this birth experience.

Fogel, Catherine Ingram, and Nancy Fugate Woods, eds. *Women's Health Care: A Comprehensive Handbook.* Thousand Oaks, CA: Sage Publications, 1995.
While all of this book enables women's self-education, in terms of self-learning for general wellness, Part III is most practical and direct. In it, the contributors consider issues of health protection and health promotion, nutritional concerns, exercise, contraceptive issues, mental health, workplace health questions, and childbearing choices. Particularly empowering to the reader, in terms of contexts of understanding in which to place their day-to-day concerns for wellness, is Chapter 11, "Health Protection and Health Promotion." This essay revolves around models of health. Its excursion into definitions of wellness and health provides a clarifying perspective for readers who know what approaches they prefer but sometimes cannot articulate names for their preferences.

Grafius, Linda C., Ed.D. *Ethics for Everyone.* Chicago: American Hospital Association, 1995.
Complete with case studies, bibliography, and resources, this book is

written for professionals such as educators, members of bioethics committees, and administrators. It addresses programs to empower health care workers, the vast majority of whom are women. It is also read with profit by women who are, in fact, in charge of the health care of their families and would be well served to have the empowering understandings which will help them negotiate that role, particularly with regard to the hospitalizations of themselves and/or their loved ones. The book provides clear explanations of the meaning and purpose of biomedical education and affords an overview of the types of topics germane to biomedical ethics. Most helpful to the reader are Chapter 4, "A Process for Ethical Thinking and Reflection," Chapter 5, "Biomedical Ethics Grand Rounds Programs," and Chapter 6, "Educational Tools." A number of the educational tools provide the reader an opportunity for gleaning by-the-way knowledge and arriving at implications which can inform their sense of control, responsibility, and self-advocacy in treatment situations.

Grant, Robert, Ph.D. *Healing the Soul of the Church: Ministers Facing Their Own Childhood Abuse and Trauma.* Burlingame, CA: Grant, 1994. This book, written directly for and for the sake of ministers in the Catholic church, can be read with profit by anyone healing from childhood abuse and trauma. The situations discussed are analogous to those experienced by people other than ministers in structures other than the church. The author points to statistics on abuse in the United States, reminding the reader that those statistics are replicated, if not surpassed, among ministers. He finds it easy to understand why the institutional church is power-driven, hierarchical, and shame based, given the number of members of the official church who are victims of abuse. "Denial, secrecy, shame, invasiveness, and adherence to false images characterize many of its most important structures" (p. 183). He finds that unrecovered victims ending up in positions of power call for others to repress or deny important life experiences and concerns in order to remain in relationship with such leadership, and he points out that those wanting to remain in clerical or religious life must adapt to this code of denial or face consequences. He deals with the results of trying to function within irrational church parameters vis-à-vis intimacy and sexuality, as well as trying to cope with the church as a "closed shop." Part I of this book offers an overview of psychological trauma. Part II shows the impact of unhealed trauma on church structures as well as on ministers.

Hicks, Karen M., ed. *Misdiagnosis: Woman as a Disease.* Allentown, PA: People's Medical Society, 1994.
This collection of essays, a number written by journalists and academics, treats most important specific topics related to women's health, from the vantage point of women's experience with relation to the health care system. Charles Inlander, author of the preface, finds that American medicine has treated the word "woman" as a medical diagnosis. The book treats issues as diverse as breast implants, reproductive questions, hysterectomies, the myth of American motherhood, HIV, and male medical bias and research consequences. The essays are clear, informative, and powerful in their poignancy as well as their humor and strength. Several of the contributors are listed in other entries in this annotated bibliography. Reading their longer works along with their essays in *Misdiagnosis* can be quite helpful, both in terms of extending information and in terms of contextualizing information.

Hoffman, Eileen, M.D. "The Emotionally Healthy Woman: Staying Well in Mind and Body." In *Our Health, Our Lives.* New York: Bantam Books, 1995.
In following through on her woman-centered insight, Hoffman includes psychological, behavioral, social, and cultural considerations in order to see a woman as a whole person. Approaching from a comprehensive environment of care, she discusses the mind-body connection and women's fight for self-esteem. She raises issues of depression as well as some of the forms of abuse which can invite it. Citing the costs of the

epidemic of violence against women in this country, Hoffman challenges the medical profession and her readers to recognize the signs of this violence and abuse. She encourages her readers to ask themselves questions pertinent to whether they are being abused. She looks at childhood sexual abuse, answers commonly asked questions, and lists resources for help. The framed reviews and checklists in this discussion are invaluable.

Hoffman, Eileen, M.D. "The Heart Disease Alert." In *Our Health, Our Lives*. New York: Bantam Books, 1995.
Pointing out that heart disease is also a women's issue, Hoffman presents clear and helpful information on CAD (coronary artery disease). Contextualizing the problem for women in descriptions of women and in past assumptions about the seriousness of their complaints, the author proceeds to data, explanations, checklists, and common questions asked by women. Explanations of each diagnostic test in this discussion give both a description of the procedure and a commentary on its accuracy for women. Hoffman closes her considerations with resources, both organizations and publications.

Hoffman, Eileen, M.D. *Our Health, Our Lives*. New York: Bantam Books, 1995.
The dedication, to Hoffman's patients, sets the tone of this book. which recognizes the bias of the medical profession and the need for learning about women's health from women's experience. Hoffman learned from her patients because she listened to them. "And when their tales were inconsistent with what I had been taught, I listened harder. Validating them, I questioned what I had been taught. This book is the story of my search for a woman-centered medicine". Within the context of a woman-centered approach, Hoffman then presents specific health issues for women with a full section of her book dedicated to mind/body connection. Uniquely helpful in her approach are specific examples from women's experiences and periodic boxes of quick step health and/or

referral information. The book is a guide to women in navigating through a health care system not designed for us.

Hoffman, Eileen, M.D. "Preventing Osteoporosis." In *Our Health, Our Lives*. New York: Bantam Books, 1995.
This discussion, Chapter 8 in Hoffman's book, is subtitled "Don't Become a Little Old Lady.. It begins with a case study and proceeds to a definition and explanation of osteoporosis. The author encourages the reader to evaluate her own risk for osteo and provides an "Are You at Risk" checklist. She discusses the benefits of calcium and includes a chart on the recommended dietary allowances. She provides a clear and concise consideration on the fact that osteo is an estrogen-connected issue and encourages the reader to sift through the issues, check through alternatives, and make decisions suitable to her personal situation. "Protect Yourself--Now and for Life" is Hoffman's opportunity to present five ways of guarding against osteoporosis. She ends her discussion with common questions asked about osteo and with resources. It is quite helpful to read this chapter of Hamilton's book in tandem with Chapter 13, "The Menopause Years: Time to Take Stock."

Hollis, Judi. *Fat Is a Family Affair*.   Center City, MN: Hazelden, 1985.
Written by a psychotherapist and a self-described recovering overeater, this book offers considerations on the family's involvement in eating disorders. It discusses family systems and co-dependency, paying attention to relationships and family messages. In presenting the isolation and loneliness connected with food obsessions, the author describes and encourages modes of honesty which help in learning to nurture self without relying on food to serve that function. The author considers anorexia and bulimia. This book can be read with greater profit alongside Joan Jacobs Brumberg, *Fasting Girls* (Harvard University Press, 1988).

Hyman, Jane Wegschieder, and Esther R. Rome, in cooperation with the Boston Women's Health Book Collective. *Sacrificing Ourselves for Love: Why Women Compromise Health and Self-Esteem . . .and How to Stop*. Freedom, CA: The Crossing Press, 1996.

This book addresses the hazards to women's health which can arise out of needs for love and acceptance. The authors' research showed them that women's willingness to risk their health for the sake of being agreeable to others eventuates from three interconnected realities: their caring attitudes, centuries of subordination, and cultural habits concerning how women ought to look, ought to behave, and ought to be treated. This three-part book treats a diversity of health issues, all connected by willingness to risk health for the sake of appeasing, being liked, finding approval, or being loved. Part I, "Trying to Look Different," addresses such issues as anorexia and bulimia, cosmetic surgery, and breast implants. It closes by offering data and suggestions on accepting self and breaking the cycle of risking health to look as one feels expected to look. Part II, "Living in Abusive Relationships," offers examples and effects of abuse, as well as suggestions for helping or getting help in escaping or ameliorating an abusive situation. It examines the myths which contribute to abuse, the social underpinnings which support it, and the failure of the legal system with regard to it. Again, the section ends with practical data and strategic advice. Part III, "Dying for Love," discusses subservience in the bedroom, sexual diseases, and the need for social change. The ending chapter in this part encourages women's choosing of self in wholesome and practical ways. This book is clear and readable, proffering helpful diagrams, charts, data reviews, and exercises. For each chapter it offers resources such as publications, films and videos, organizations, hot lines, and audio cassettes.

Johnson, Karen, M.D., and Tom Ferguson, M.D. *Trusting Ourselves: The Sourcebook on Psychology for Women*. New York: The Atlantic Monthly Press, 1990.

This clear and readable volume is presented in four parts. Part I, "A

Summary of the Psychology of Women," offers a historical as well as a contemporary perspective which creates a context for the professional and non-professional alike. It is a particularly helpful way for the reader to get a sense of things. Part II, "Relationships: The Fulcrum of Women's Psychology," not only presents discussion on specific relationships, but also provides a sense of where women's psychology as a field of consideration has grown since the work of Gilligan. Part III, "Signs and Symptoms: Common Psychological Concerns," considers such issues as self-esteem, depression, anxiety, sexuality, alcohol, eating disorders, and abuse and violence. Part IV, "Making Changes," is the most immediately practical section of this work. Chapter 13, "Taking Your Own History" has a clear and helpful approach, including genogram considerations, as well as data and outlines. Perhaps most important for readers looking for assistance is Chapter 14, "Using Professional Assistance." Its information and advice on finding a psychiatrist is transferable to finding help from any therapeutic professional and provides the reader a sense of her own power in the process. The epilogue is a highly encouraging understanding and appreciation of the integration of women's experience into descriptions of psychological health, and of the strength, courage, and resourcefulness of women.

Kahn, Ada P., and Linda Hughes Holt, M.D. *Midlife Health: Every Woman's Guide to Feeling Good.* New York: Facts on File, 1987.
At the time of their writing of this book the authors were surprised to find that many gynecology textbooks contained only one chapter concerning menopause, and that generally placed right before the chapter on senility. Concerned because one third of women's lifespan is now in the postmenopausal years, they sent questionnaires to 2,000 women between the ages of 45 and 60. Because they summarize the respondents' answers throughout their book, the authors consider this work to be a conversation among women. This work is a guidebook combining medical and self-help information presented in a practicable manner. It

aims at helping women to utilize the medical care system not only wisely but economically, as it attempts to prepare them for health in midlife and beyond. Three specific aids beyond the data and dynamics of this book are the glossary, the bibliography, and the appendix, which contains the original questionnaire. This book is read with profit in conjunction with Gail Sheehy's *The Silent Passage* (Random House, 1992).

Kurtz, Ron. *Body-Centered Psychotherapy: The Hakomi Method.* Mendocino, CA: LifeRhythm, 1990.

Pointing out the contemporary situation as a time for holists and people who love diversity, the author presents the Hakomi method of Body/Mind Therapy as grounded in principles for shifting paradigms. He offers Hakomi as a nonviolent psychotherapy, one that evokes the wisdom and the healing power in each. Hakomi, a Hopi Indian word, translates as "How do you stand in relation to these many realities?" Some Hakomi concepts, such as, gentleness, compassion, and mindfulness, originate in Taoism and Buddhism. Kurtz combines these with a sense of the organic integration of matter, energy, and environment, as well as with the contributions of Gestalt, Bioenergetics, and other body-based therapies. The book has a clarity and a humor which invite the reader to reflect upon insights while understanding the author's principles and approach. The quotations opening each chapter, as well as the diagrams, columns, and examples, make that understanding easy.

Lutter, Judy Mahle, and Lynn Jaffee of the Melpomene Institute for Women's Health Research. *The Bodywise Woman.* Champaign, IL: Human Kinetics, 1996.

This second edition of *The Bodywise Woman*, revised and broadened, has been updated in terms of research and has added visual extras such as sidebars, photos, tables, figures, and personal profiles. It presents an easy to read format with effective routes for finding information. Divided into seven chapters, the book presents an excellent combination of history, questions of body image, encouragement and advice, exercise during pregnancy, and aging and ongoing activity. Threaded through the text are specific considerations such as eating disorders, nutritional facts, weight tables, menstrual questions and hormone replacement, and advice on honoring one's own body in making decisions about exercise and health. It contextualizes questions and issues in the larger social and political realm, taking into consideration Title IX legislation and the decline of women coaches since that legal enactment. The approach in this book is clearly that of women's whole health across the lifespan. The book is well read in conjunction with Carol Gilligan, Janie Victoria Ward, and Jill McLean Taylor, *Mapping the Moral Domain* (Harvard University Press, 1988), and Patricia Vertinsky, *The Eternally Wounded Woman* (Manchester University Press, 1990).

Nicarthy, Ginny, Naomi Gottlieb, and Sandra Hoffman. *You Don't Have to Take It: A Woman's Guide to Confronting Emotional Abuse at Work.* Seattle, WA: Seal Press, 1993.
Seeking to raise awareness of workplace abuse of women and to offer women alternatives in confronting that abuse, the authors begin and end with an understanding of the larger social context enabling workplace abuse. Having noticed the importance of paid work in women's lives, they experienced disappointment in how little attention has been paid to women's problems on the job. Focus groups and personal interviews provide the primary information of this book. Considerations include the power of naming abuse, understanding oneself within the situation, strategizing for action, and joining others in action. Sexual harassment is treated as a particular category of emotional abuse. The layout of this book, its clarity, and its helpful exercises provide the reader a chance for reflectivity and for self-recognition while, entertaining the larger picture.

Samuelson, Michael H. *Action Plans for Personal Stress Management: Turning Challenges into Opportunities.* Ann Arbor, MI: The National Center for Health Promotion, 1991.

While this work does not attend specifically to women's health and is, in fact, an approach for people in the business world, it provides helpful information as well as insights. Its introduction sets the context by providing data, goals, and possible benefits. Each chapter is highly practical, offering self-assessment opportunities, diagrams/graphics, and possibilities for action plans. One advantage of this book, in fact, is the ongoing sense, as well as built-in skills presentation, of the action plan as a mode of approach and as a tool for accomplishment. Most readers will find the worksheets a primary plus in this book.

Schaefer, Charles E., Ph.D., and Theresa DiGeronimo, M.Ed. *How to Talk to Your Kids About Really Important Things*. San Francisco: Jossey-Bass, 1994.
Aware that a child's questions concerning daily life can take parents by surprise, Schaefer and DiGeronimo encourage parents in finding what they need in order to talk with their children and answer their difficult questions. Through vignettes and sample conversations, the authors provide practical advice and guidance pertaining to a range of issues. In Part I, " Major Crises and Big Family Changes," they discuss such issues as adoption, death, family changes, doctor and dentist visits, moving, an alcoholic parent, and hospital stays. In Part II, "Concerns of Youth," they offer guidance on questions of drug abuse, HIV/AIDS, homosexuality, prejudice, risk taking and failure, sexual abuse, television and other media, violence, and war.

Scully, Diana. *Men Who Control Women's Health: The Miseducation of Obstetrician-Gynecologists*. Boston: Houghton Mifflin, 1980.
Providing a helpful glossary of medical terms and a set of resources on books, newsletters, and films, this book provides a historical tone and sweep which can be a contextualizing influence in understanding current questions. The author, a sociologist, studied surgical training and discovered attitudes which helped to explain the increase in obstetric and gynecologic surgery. She also discovered attitudes and professional goals

that were at variance with women's health care needs. While some things have changed since the date of this work's publication, the presentation of tones and attitudes, as well as data, affords the reader an opportunity to frame her questions so that she may see where things have not yet changed. In Chapter 1, "The Problem," the author is able to recognize health care in the United States as a system in crisis, as well as a monopoly. From that framework, she can consider sexism in medicine. She locates issues of control and, though she weaves strategies throughout her text, she devotes her final chapter to "Strategies for Change."

Sheehy, Gail. *New Passages: Mapping Your Life Across Time.* New York: Random House, 1995.

This book deals primarily with middle life, that is, the years of the mid-forties to mid-sixties. It is a book which Sheehy was researching when she stopped to write *The Silent Passage*, a necessary detour on her way to finishing this work. *New Passages* presents, in a thematic manner, the surprise and rebirth possibilities of middle life, possibilities that did not fit within former maps of youth and age. Sheehy found in her explorations that the second half of contemporary adult life can be an exhilarating starting over. She discovered that it is a progress story rather than a decline, that people can look forward to living decades longer than formerly and to functioning well during that time. Thus, she redefines the gift of midlife. The pictorial map on the inside covers of the book outlines the matter of the text: Provisional Adulthood: 18-30, First Adulthood: 30-45, and Second Adulthood: 45-85+. Placed on that map are some of the major insights with which she deals in her chapters, such as male "menopause," meaning crisis, the "sexual diamond," active risk-taking, and mature love. Sheehy's Part Six, "Passage to the Age of Integrity," is well read alongside Wendy Lustbader and Nancy Hodyman, *Taking Care of Aging Family Members: A Practical Guide* (The Free Press, 1994).

Sheehy, Gail. *The Silent Passage*. New York: Random House, 1992.
The author names two wellsprings for this book: her own ignorance and the overwhelming response to an article of hers breaking the taboo about menopause. Aware of her own experience of lack of ready information concerning menopause, quite different from the wealth of ready information about pregnancy, Sheehy committed herself to listening to women to record their experiences with this change of life. She hoped their stories would be catalytic for honest discussions. She sought women from varied geographies, races, and classes, in all interviewing more than one hundred women in different stages of menopause. She gleaned standard medical information as well as information from allied fields. Then, she consulted scholars of sociology, anthropology, history, and primate research. Sheehy's book contains four sections: "The Need to Know and the Fear of Knowing," "The Perimenopause Panic," "The Menopause Gateway," and "Coalescence". Her postscript is a warm and lovely piece of prose, sharing not only a part of her story but also her way of seeing an important life event for women.

Shreve, Anita. *Women Together, Women Alone: The Legacy of the Consciousness-Raising Movement.* New York: Viking Penguin, 1989.
Presenting a history of consciousness-raising groups in the United States, Shreve points out that images of the middle-class household, with a woman primarily as the support to her husband and children, is a relatively recent phenomenon. She takes the reader through the time of Rosie the Riveter into the time of the pink-collar workforce. She shows the isolation of women in their homes previous to the 1960s and points out feminist writings which invited consciousness-raising groups into being. Shreve is clear that consciousness-raising groups provided women who participated with an invaluable set of skills: fluency; clarity; respect, trust, and love for other women; support for experience; and insight. Placing the first formal introduction of consciousness-raising into the Women's Movement on Thanksgiving Day, 1968, Shreve notes that times have changed, and she wonders what happened to those women

who participated in CR (consciousness-raising) groups. She spent from 1986 to 1988 finding out by interviewing 65 women, between the ages of 34 and 55 years, who had belonged to such groups. Most of the women have children, and most are in the paid workforce. These women, a barometer of the CR legacy, show that women are once again isolated, not in the same way they were in the 1960s but in ways which are still inhibiting. Their isolation comes mainly from trying to stay afloat, juggling work and family obligations, dealing with child care issues, being single parents, competing in the workplace, being part of the "sandwich" generation, and aging. They find themselves facing moral dilemmas over such issues as women exploiting women and the feminization of poverty. There is a sense that women don't have each other anymore. The chapters in this book are insightful and challenging, and the appendix, "Suggested Topics for Consciousness-Raising," a practical aid.

Simeone, Angela. *Academic Women: Working Towards Equality.* South Hadley, MA: Bergin and Garvey, 1987.
With a foreword by Jesse Barnard, this work discusses the effects of moves to achieve equality for women in the field of higher education. It points out the progress achieved since the 1964 publication of Barnard's book *Academic Women.* Simeone concludes that improvements with regard to antidiscrimination policy and institutional support for women have been made in part because of the organization and networking of women faculty on their own behalf. The chapters of this book consider such issues as career choice; that is, formal status measured by salary, rank, and tenure, as well as roles; such as teacher and researcher. They also discuss marital status, family issues, and relationships among women faculty. This book is well read alongside Nadyna Aisenberg and Mona Harrington's *Women of Academe* (University of Massachusetts Press, 1988), providing the reader an examination of similarities and dissimilarities of approach and conclusions. The comparison also aids the reader in her construction of

the history of the questions, bringing a sense of how long they have been formally posed.

Travis, John W., M.D., and Meryn G. Callander. *Wellness for Helping Professionals: Creating Compassionate Cultures*. Mill Valley, CA: Wellness Associates Publications, 1990.
With a foreword by Larry Dossey, this information/workbook addresses its topic from three vantage points: heart, head, and hands. This is clearly an approach quite appropriate for helping professionals. The contents and the contents overview in the beginning pages lay out the scope of the book through the use of graphic representations. The heart component, Part I, "Personal Journey," invites the readers to consciously engage in their own personal process so that they might integrate the conceptual component of wellness. The authors encourage the readers by sharing portions of their own personal journeys. The matter of Part II, "Conceptual Understanding," or head, contrasts the consciousness of the "Discountability Paradigm" with that of "Accountability," discussing these from the vantage points of personal life, professional practice, and planetary considerations. It provides a series of learning modules which are not only readable but also easily digested so that the reader is free to sift and reflect. Hands, or Part III, "Practical Applications," provides not only skills for program designing but also aids for developing approaches to conflict resolution. The data, checklists, and worksheets in this section are eminently useful and useable. Anyone who has asked herself, "Who heals the healer?" is likely to find profit in this book.

Travis, John W., M.D., and Regina Sara Ryan. *Wellness Workbook*. Second edition. Berkeley, CA: Ten Speed Press, 1988.
While this book does not specifically address women's health as such, it does present helpful information, clear and useful review diagrams, and empowering worksheets. Its whole systems approach considers wellness, rather than illness care, perceiving this through the lenses of managing the forms of energy moving in and out of one's body. The

book contains twelve chapters, each of which discusses one of the twelve forms of energy presented by the authors. "The Wellness Index," offered immediately after the introduction to this workbook, is an effective self-assessment through which the reader can focus personal direction in attending to the ensuing chapters. The original edition of this book was published in 1981, just as the discussions among quantum mechanics, philosophy, religion, and more general transformational concerns were coming into public view. The appendices present practical information on music and on journaling.

Verbrugge, Martha H. "Knowledge and Power: Health and Physical Education for Women in America." In Rima D. Apple, ed., *Women, Health and Medicine in America: A Historical Handbook*. New York: Garland, 1990.

Alerting the reader to the insight that both health education and physical education are not neutral bodies of data, the author encourages noticing hidden curricula in each. She not only traces historical points from nineteenth century caveats through Title IX legislation but also raises the dual questions of the relationships between health and physical education and gender socialization and the possible synergy between women's physical freedom and their social empowerment. She points to the connections between women's legal and cultural gains and physical liberation. In her conclusions, Verbrugge raises calls for further research on crucial questions pertinent to relationships among health education, physical activities, and female socialization, naming several areas worthy of particular attention: a broadened scope of histories of physical education in schools; an increased knowledge concerning physical education in gymnasia, supervised playgrounds, and recreational clubs; and study of the roles of women's voluntary organizations. With regard to both health education and physical education, Verbrugge calls for more research about the formulation, dissemination, and effects of who educated women to health, with what goals, employing what models of health, and using what information and programs. She also seeks knowledge from a focus on the numerous women who provided health and physical education, including teachers, college professors, coaches, social workers, and public health nurses.

Weed, Susan S. *Menopausal Years the Wise Woman Way.* Woodstock, NY: Ash Tree, 1992.
Written in popular style, this treatment of menopause encourages women to pay attention to the messages of their own bodies. Having spent three years interviewing women on their experience of menopause, the author found their accounts quite different from many published ones. Couched in crone imagery, with advice and understanding provided by "Grandmother Growth," the book explains by providing data, supports by suggesting practical dynamics, informs by giving explanations of herbal remedies, and provides direction for further reading by including references and resources. The dynamic of this book, written in three chapters, is a rhythmic pattern of the data/issues considered in the respective chapter, references and resources, herbal allies, and ritual interlude. The dynamic itself models menopause as a new life integration.

Witkin, Dr. Georgia. *The Truth About Women: Fighting the Fourteen Devastating Myths That Hold Women Back.* New York: Viking, 1995.
With a powerful preface, the author places her direction squarely before the reader's eyes. Women don't love men who hate them, are not lacking mechanical aptitude, and are not crazed when premenstrual. She places the reasons for myths and psychobabble in three among many reasons: myths are dramatic, myths are convenient, and myths are camouflage. Deciding that the cost of myths, as she describes them, is too high, Witkin feels assured that women are ready to give up the myths and see new truth. Her chapters are laid out in a pattern. The author states the myth, briefly naming correlates. Then she considers, "Who Believes It?," followed by "The Truth" and "How to Use the Truth." Each chapter ends with a neatly outlined, specifically practical, boxed presentation on "Countering the Myth." The data and strategies in this book are garnered

from four sources: clinical interviews, local surveys, a national computer-based survey, and in-depth interviews. This book provides strategies for women demanding equitable costs in health care, particularly as health care reform evolves.

Wolin, Steven J., M.D., and Sybil Wolin, Ph.D. *The Resilient Self: How Survivors of Troubled Families Rise Above Adversity.* New York: Villard Books, 1994.

Written from the proactive stance of building upon innate or acquired strengths, this book provides a clearly written and insightful treatment of the clusters of resiliencies typical of survivors of troubled families as they struggle with adversity.Writing with the understanding which is a product of years of research and clinical experience, the Wolins identify seven resiliencies around which they build their Challenge Model. By placing their experience and knowledge into the hands of survivors, the Wolins teach and encourage a reflective sifting which can distinguish, without ignoring, the pain of a troubled childhood from the courage, strength, heart, and risk-taking capabilities which negotiating that childhood brought to the fore. The seven resiliencies named by the authors are insight, independence, relationships, initiative, creativity, humor, and morality.

COSTS AND BENEFITS

INTRODUCTION

Over the past three decades, there have been major changes in religious, philosophical, psychological, and biological understandings, with concomitant changes in belief systems. Philosophically absolutist and biologically deterministic views have been replaced by understandings that the actual determinants of women's health are, in fact, social and economic. While these changes in thought and understanding are relatively new, the behaviors for which they call are, by and large, still the old ones. Changes in understanding have not yet become changes in appropriate access and treatment for women. Even where women have the financial wherewithal to obtain health care, the research appropriate to specifically female health and the cultural change necessary for implementing appropriate approaches lag behind the discoveries.

Women's traditional roles have substantially limited their access to education and to health care, at the same time that their contributions to any nation's and the world's health have been overlooked. Public health agencies, on an international level, have become aware that the health of a nation's women is ultimately a clear indicator of the health of that nation. The debilitating disease of poverty, which affects two thirds of women on a global level, shows itself in discrete physical symptoms such as anemia, malnutrition, fatigue, increased susceptibility to invasive infections, and ultimately premature death. Gender bias as well as resource allocation, including these elements in the developed countries, make health care for women unavailable and/or unaffordable to many of them. Women's lack of ownership of the world's property and the means of production, as well as their sexually defined roles and status, has left them at high risk of health problems including those created by violence and abuse against them. Ultimately, the costs to the household of humanity of not attending to women's whole health across the lifespan is enormous, not only in monetary terms but also in terms of human dignity, relationships, productivity, creativity, and quality. These last, perhaps least clearly seen, are, over the long haul, most costly to the human community.

Much of this bibliography has already, at least indirectly, pointed out the implicate costs and benefits of fostering women's whole health. This introduction makes a brief note about what I choose to call good beginnings and good endings with regard to women's health across the lifespan. Thus, a few words about adolescents' and elderly women's health, and these from the perspective of the United States system.

Violence against and abuse of women remains a prime women's health issue in the United States. While one might not immediately see all of the costs to health care, they exist. The cost to taxpayers in terms of legislation, emergency care, government programs for the abused and the abuser, and court costs may sit "on the books" elsewhere than in the health care system, but they are costs nonetheless. No "books" can itemize the cost in shattered lives, loss of esteem, fractured egos, self-imposed restrictions, and the cost to productivity of these. Both younger and older women suffer abuse, at least, if not more than, other segments of the female population. Societal beliefs as well as reporting procedures result in underreporting the number of cases which actually exist. If violence against women were properly attended to, and if the health care system were better able to assess this problem during routine health exams, monies presently spent in actual health care costs resulting from violence against women could be freed for other health care use. Lack of knowledge on the part of many health professionals in terms of assessing other factors before a severe episode, as well as reluctance to broach the subject, increase costs while decreasing benefits of present treatment.

The health care community has made large strides, however, in other aspects of preventive medicine. Since the American Medical Association's proposal for annual physical exams in 1922, and its endorsement in 1983, effective interventions addressing personal health practices have led to reductions in incidence and severity of some diseases and disabilities. Education, both at the level of public awareness and at the level of healing professionals' understanding their educative function, has increased patient/clinician shared decision making and fostered health from a more proactive perspective than the mere absence of disease. The immediate costs may appear higher; however, the benefits are likely to be more immediate, and the costs over the long haul should be less.

In adolescent years, ages 13-19, while girls are negotiating both physical and emotional transitions into womanhood, homicide is among the leading causes of death, and sexual abuse is among the leading causes of illness for them. Among young women 15-24 years of age homicide is the second largest health issue, with suicide first. Both are many times related to exposure to violence. These problems, in terms of frequency, are followed by drugs, alcohol, and sexual issues (unsafe sex).

In the United States two thirds of minimum wage workers are women, and over one fifth of women raising families alone are below the poverty level. Women facing, or in, retirement are an excellent case in point for considering costs and benefits, both to the women themselves and to the society in which they live. By and large, Social Security benefits to women are minimal, for any number of reasons, including women's employment part-time and pink collar, or low paid in sectors other than pink collar; and as interrupted for the sake of childbearing/rearing and caretaking of the health of family members, in particular disabled ones. This latter has become an even more crucial consideration, given the experience of the sandwich generation, which has been juggling the care of two generations, their children and their parents. Access to health care for themselves as well as for their parents is an economic hardship, not only in monetary but, in larger personal, relational, and health terms. Housing as a health and economic issue for older women, as well as nutrition, functional ability, greater vulnerability to abuse, alcoholism, and polypharmacy issues, needs consideration in a way not understood previously. Outmoded beliefs concerning the aging process, especially with regard to women, have left the health care system with limited expertise. The limited perspective of such beliefs can result in failure to see situations amenable to treatment, labeling these as the inevitable consequences of aging.

The books in this set of annotations have a reasonably large representation among women and work questions. These books tend to point to the economy of women and work, that is, the health costs and benefits, not just with regard to concrete disease risks in certain jobs or job sites but also in relation to the overall consequences of women's overwork and underpay. Even the rushed pace of the work environment cuts into the possible benefits of preventive and lifestyle health efforts. Issues of the glass ceiling, for instance, not only create stress problems but also leave no time for attending to preventive as well as disease issues. Any consideration of women and work involves the costs and benefits, the total *oeconomia*, of heath care and health care reform, since women's largest health issue is overload of work and lack of access to care . The present world economy demands such unpaid for and unfairly paid for work on the part of women, that in impacting their health, it ultimately impacts the health of all related to them. In short, it impacts global health. In this instance, equity matters not simply as a matter of principle and justice, but as a matter of good health.

Shifts in national budgetary priorities as well as shifts in health care management systems are increasingly called for. There is an unconscionable cost to any country in the final consequences of either improper or insufficient care for 52% of its population.

ANNOTATIONS

Albelda, Randy, and Chris Tilly. *Glass Ceilings and Bottomless Pits: Women's Work, Women's Poverty.* Boston: South End Press, 1997.
The female executive and the welfare mother may appear to be worlds apart, but they share some things in common: job discrimination, lower pay than men, and primary responsibility for the unpaid work of caring for their children. This book offers an analysis of the economic and social

realities faced by women across class lines in the United States. Clear and readable and filled with supporting data, this work provides an explanation of the impact of rapid economic changes and rapid cultural changes in the United States in the past fifty years. These changes have caused increasing pressure on families and have left single mothers farther and farther behind. The authors consider how the discussion around women's issues has been manipulated to separate women of upper and middle classes from their poorer sisters. They examine the results of public policies, and they propose concrete strategies for transforming policies to provide real support for families and to secure women's economic equality. This book is enriched by reading with Mayra Buvinic and SallyW. Yudelman, *Women, Poverty and Progress in the Third World* (The Foreign Policy Association, 1989).

Bergman, Barbara A. *The Economic Emergence of Women.* New York: Basic Books, 1986.

Arguing that contemporary changes show a concrete difference from centuries-old sex roles, Bergman analyzes the questions and needs created by participation of women in American economy, that is, in its paid labor force. She discusses social changes and gender differences in the workplace, including wage discrepancies, affirmative action, and gender discrimination. Since these affect family, household, economy, and national policy agenda, Bergman proposes changed policies to reflect these realities. Her proposals regarding movements against discrimination and harassment, creation and enforcement of relevant laws, recognition and policies with regard to comparable worth, adoption of child care and child support policies, and encouragement of shifts in cultural attitudes remain live questions for working women, particularly for those in the health care fields.

Briles, Judith. *GenderTraps: Conquering Confrontophobia, Toxic Bosses, and Other Land Mines at Work.* New York: McGraw-Hill, 1996.

The author of this book is a speaker, a researcher of women, and a consultant. Speaking with over 5,000 women, sending out 5,000 questionnaires, processing 1,270 written survey responses, and interviewing 130 respondents, she arrives at conclusions similar to those of the survey conducted by the Women's Bureau of the U.S. Department of Labor. The similarities of response across work places from jailhouse to secretarial pool to management office to operating room are such that the author concludes that GenderTraps experiences are transposable to many work environments. She lists, then discusses in detail, the ten most common GenderTraps in the workplace. Surprisingly enough, sexual harassment and the glass ceiling take a back seat to such issues as prejudice, sabotage, management chaos, pay inequities, balancing family and work, and misuse of power. This book offers the voices and personal stories of workers, as well as the data and strategies provided by its author. It is clearly written, with graphically boxed definitions and reminders, and includes questionnaires and diagrams. The afterword and appendix, "The Workplace Trap Survey," provide the reader, respectively, with a sense of the dream of the author and the original survey, in context, from which this book arose.

Campbell, Alastair. *Health as Liberation: Medicine, Theology and the Quest for Justice.* Cleveland, OH: The Pilgrim Press, 1995.
Based on the Tuohy lectures given at John Carroll University in 1994, this work deals ultimately with *oeconomia*. Seeing from the vantage point of liberation thinking and practice, and describing health as liberation, the author listens to many voices of illness and pays attention to the social structures which can frustrate or encourage health. While this work does not specifically regard women and health, nor the financial costs and benefits connected with that question, it provides helpful insight in enlightening directions. The chapter on "Power and Powerlessness in Health Care" does consider the health care crisis in the United States, pointing out the inequity of the burden of ill health within that population. Chapter 5, "What Price Liberation? The Quest for

Justice," reframes the questions from a theologico-ethical framework. Read side by side with Jean Achterberg's *Woman as Healer* (Shambala, 1990), particularly her work on healing and the healing system, in Chapter 17, this work can raise new questions and new perspectives with regard to the ultimate economy of women and health.

Dimond, Margaret. "Older Women's Health." In Catherine Ingram Fogel and Nancy Fugate Woods, eds., *Women's Health Care: A Comprehensive Handbook.* Thousand Oaks, CA: Sage Publications, 1995.

When one looks at the demographic information with regard to aging women, the biopsychosocial aspects of their aging, and the political and economic forces affecting older women's lives, there are implicate costs and benefits in dealing well with women's health issues during this part of their lifespan. Between 1990 and 2050, it is projected that the population over 65 years of age will increase by 117% while the number of those over 85 will quadruple, the largest percentage of these being women. The combination of poverty and chronic disease for these women, intensified among women in underrepresented ethnic groups, makes it clear that most of the issues of aging will, in fact, be women's issues. Because older women with better educational and financial resources will likely have more options for remaining more actively engaged in life, it is to the overall benefit of a nation to tend to the long-term costs, both human and financial, which will accrue to poverty and ill health among older women. Even in the face of Medicare and Medicaid in the United States, there are barriers to the receipt of good health care by women. Inequities in women's earnings, inequities in Social Security benefits, and statistics confirming the rising percentage of older women in the population are not being sufficiently addressed in public policies affecting aging women, or in research. This essay contextualizes the costs/benefits question within the multiple issues of older women's health.

Eisler, Riane. *Sacred Pleasure: Sex, Myth, and the Politics of the Body*.
    San Francisco: Harper, 1996.
    This book, which points to a new integration of the sexual, the spiritual,
    and the social, ultimately envisions a new economy, that is, new ways of
    relating for the good of the whole household of humankind. The author
    connects her considerations with what she calls the "economics of
    domination," as distinct and different from the "economics of
    partnership." Eisler's Part 1, "How Did We Get Here?," treats a wide-
    ranging socio-cultural history of sex. "Where Are We and Where Do We
    Go from Here?" deals with transformational issues presented through
    critical thinking, understanding, sifting, and changing. The whole of this
    second part comes together in Chapters 17, 18, and 19, where Eisler
    makes her case for a real transformation which not only redefines politics
    and economics but brings the human back to the creative adventure in a
    totally new way. "The Dominator and Partnership Models" provided
    after Chapter 19 are quite helpful and reminiscent of Eisler's previous
    two books, *The Chalice and the Blade* (1987), and *The Partnership
    Way* (1990).

Evans, Sara M., and Barbara J. Nelson. *Wage Justice: Comparable Worth
    and the Paradox of Technocratic Reform*. Chicago: University of
    Chicago Press, 1989.
    This book deals with the "equal pay for equal work" concept of the
    1960s, which moved through the 1970s as "comparable worth." Evans
    and Nelson discuss this concept as it appears in the experience of the
    state of Minnesota. Minnesota was among state leaders when it passed
    pay equity acts adapted from the theory of comparable worth at the state
    level in 1982 and at the local level in 1984. Minnesota's efforts have
    proceeded farther than those of other states. The authors of *Wage Justice*
    deal with the complexities in creating and implementing comparable
    worth policies, which they consider to have been virtually ignored in
    public and scholarly debate. They explore the practical question of how
    well comparable worth works, and they focus on the broader theoretical

issues the concept raises. This book aims at pointing out the consequences of comparable worth policy for individuals, for organizations, and for society in general. While meeting their aims the authors discuss paradoxes of distributive justice. They consider horizontal justice in a vertical-that is, hierarchical-world. They point out the technocratic reform and democratic values revealed by implementation of comparable worth. The historical context as well as the clear sifting of the issues provided by this book, as well as the appendices, speak to dilemmas of contemporary democracy.

Fields, Richard, Ph.D. "Drugs/Alcohol: The Modern Disease of Our American Society." In *Drugs in Perspective*. Madison, WI: Brown and Benchmark, 1995.

In this eleventh chapter of his book, Fields deals with changes in health care reform while considering the larger societal issues affecting alcoholism and other drug addiction. In the economy of health care, approximately 70% of federal monies put aside for tending to the nation's drug problem are being spent on reducing the supply of drugs in the United States. This supply side expenditure has created a neglect of funding for demand side programs for prevention, intervention, and treatment. There have been cuts in block grant programs for states, cuts in the Department of Education's "drug free" schools program, and shifts of monies to more centralized agencies. Funding cuts and shifts, as well as lacks in cooperation among diverse perspectives in dealing with alcohol/drug problems and lack of cooperation between drug/alcohol and mental health/psychiatric fields, compound the problems of tending to the thousands of those who are waiting to enter publicly funded treatment. Beyond the two systemic problems mentioned above, a third systemic problem affecting the ultimate costs of the alcohol/drug health issue is what still remains the inequity of treatment for people of color. Fields also points toward the ultimate costs accruing from the failure of the U.S. educational system and to those accruing from socioeconomic inequities discouraging the underclass.

Fox, Mary Frank, and Sharlene Hess-Biber. *Women at Work*. Palo Alto,
CA: Mayfield, 1984.

Particularly helpful in its tables, figures, and bibliography, this social
scientific study provides a preindustrial to contemporary history of
women and work in the United States. Fox and Hess-Biber, in pointing
up the secondary status of women in the workforce, provide clear
understandings of sex segregation, changes in work roles, and women's
participation in paid labor, as well as the functions, both social and
economic, of work in U.S. culture. The authors are concretely aware of
the biases of male-centered work studies previous to their publication.
In the face of rising numbers of women in the paid labor force of the
United States-almost half-and the major percentage of these women
employed at minimum wage level, the understandings provided by Fox
and Hess-Biber become all the more timely.

Groneman, Carol, and Mary Beth Norton, eds. *"To Toil the Livelong
Day": America's Women at Work, 1780-1980*. Ithaca, NY: Cornell
University Press, 1987.

This book is a collection of historical and scholarly essays on women and
work. Chronologically arranged, it includes a number of facets of
importance in each historical period it considers, including studies of
agricultural workers in the 1870-1920 period and the Women's Bureau
of the United Automobile Workers in the 1940-1980s period. Two
specifically helpful aspects are that a good number of the essays consider
race, ethnicity, and class issues and that the historical overlap of periods
tends to draw the threads of continuity among them. The description of
a continuum of paid and unpaid women's labor shows the need for new
models of women's work. This last consideration can be particularly
helpful now as women face more and heavier expectations to provide
unpaid health care for those for whom the health system provides fewer
and more brief services.

Jacobson, Jodi. "Women's Health: The Price of Poverty." In Marge

Koblinsky, Jill Gay, and Judith Timyan, eds., *The Health of Women: A Global Perpective*. Boulder, CO: Westview, 1993.

In this essay, Jacobson describes the disease of poverty. She points out that two out of three women suffer from this debilitating condition, which exhibits common symptoms, such as chronic anemia, malnutrition, and severe fatigue. She finds this disease communicated from mother to child, with markedly higher transmission rates among females than among males. The fact is that macroeconomic policies that are increasing inequality in the United States are the same ones generating a wider rift between developed and underdeveloped countries. In face of this situation, not only are women suffering greater lack of health, but they also are lacking access to treatment for these problems. This is difficult to understand when simple technology and simple preventive measures could alleviate these situations.

Jarvik, Lissy, M.D., Ph.D., and Gary Small, M.D. *ParentCare: Common sense for Adult Children*. New York: Crown, 1988.

This guidebook for the sandwich generation is replete with data and advice for those caught between caring for their children and caring for their parents. Until the end of the twentieth century the parenting cycle was a case of being raised by one's parents, becoming old enough to take care of oneself, and then raising one's own children. Not so long ago, 60 was considered "old age." Advances in medicine, technology, and living conditions have provided longer life. Also, adults have opted to have children later in life than was previously customary. The sandwich generation finds itself faced with two generations competing for its attention. Parenting aging parents has important differences from parenting young children, and it is these differences and the concomitant needs which *ParentCare* addresses. In effect, the larger responsibility falls upon women. Upper-income families are likely to hire caregivers and provide their parents separate housing until, eventually, extended care in outside facilities is necessary. For those without income or skills, the situation is even more difficult. In any case, the stress engendered in the ongoing tending may invite disease and family disruption. This book is multifaceted in approaching its concerns and strategies from the point of view of both the cared for and the caregiver. The appendices are quite practical and immediately useful: Appendix 1, "Some Common Health Problems," Appendix 2, "What Can You Do If Your Parent Has Alzheimer Disease?," Appendix 3, "Who's Who in Health Care," Appendix 4, "Side Effects of Antidepressants," Appendix 5, "Durable Power of Attorney," Appendix 6, "The Living Will," and Appendix 7, "Other Resources."

Kaminer, Wendy. *Women Volunteering: The Pleasure, Pain and Politics of Unpaid Work From 1830 to the Present.* Garden City, NY: Anchor Press/Doubleday, 1984.

Discussing the meaning of women's experience as volunteers, Kaminer begins her book with a history of female volunteers but stresses experience contemporary with the book's publication date. She does this by drawing on interviews with women committed to volunteer work, questioning their motives and feelings and reflecting upon their responses in light of attitudes about women and work in the 1970s and 1980s. Her interviewees represent a wide variety of ages, life situations, types of employment, and reasons for volunteering. The beauty of this book is in its underlying understanding of work, not to be confused with paid labor only. Though it is not the matter of this book, the reader may wonder what happens when women are "volunteered."

Levine, Susan. *Labor's True Woman: Carpet Weavers, Industrialization, and Labor Reform in the Gilded Age.* Philadelphia: Temple University Press, 1984.

By 1880 women were 18% of the paid labor force, not a sufficient percentage to be considered major players in the post Civil War industrial transformation. In fact, among those women in the paid labor force the larger number were domestic servants. Most studies, suggesting that women worked only out of dire necessity, have reinforced the public/private split, paying little attention to the home and work dynamic in the Gilded Age of industrialization. Neither did they pay attention to women's roles in working-class communities. Newer studies, including studies in women's history, have tended to skip over the late nineteenth century, leaving a gap in United States labor history and hiding women in discussions of domesticity. This work is a study of working-class women in the world of the Gilded Age. It shows that women workers in the United States, by the 1880s, were a fact of life, growing to 20% of the paid labor force by 1910. The book looks closely at the experience of one group, New York State and Philadelphia carpet weavers. It addresses several gaps, showing that the power loom of the 1870s called for unskilled and semi-skilled workers, who, in fact, were young women, to replace skilled craftsmen. The book considers their strike, supported by the Knights of Labor, pointing out that women as wage earners had a place. However, organized labor's commitment to equal rights for these women was in tension, if not clash, with notions of domesticity and women's sphere. Chapter 6, "Limits of Labor Ideology: Equal Rights and Domesticity in the Labor Movement," shows this tension. Alice Kessler-Harris' *Out to Work* (Oxford University Press, 1982) and Elizabeth Anne Payne's *Reform, Labor, and Feminism* (University of Illinois Press, 1988), are good companions to this book. The issues of percentages of female wage earners, expectations concerning women's sphere, and the commitment of organized labor, in particular health care service labor to women, are still pressing.

Lustbader, Wendy, and Nancy R. Hooyman. *Taking Care of Aging Family Members: A Practical Guide.* Revised and expanded edition. New York: The Free Press, 1994.

The illustrations, checklists, charts, forms, suggested resources, and reminders in this volume are invaluable aids in making the reading manageable and for getting about the business of extending good care. This book offers families much needed information for care of their aging members as well as for care of their own needs. It can be read by professionals, by volunteers, and by students in the healing professions as well as by family members. The initial five chapters look over the emotional territory of caring for aging family members, discussing stresses, dynamics between partners, siblings' attempts to share the care, and special considerations for atypical families. Other chapters suggest methods of promoting collaborative efforts, exploring publicly funded programs, finding long-term care services, and extending family caregiving into the aging person's nursing home experience. This book employs a wide net for describing family and uses a gender-inclusive approach by alternating female and male pronouns. Its detailed index is particularly helpful. This book is an excellent companion to Lissy Jarvik and Gary Small, *ParentCare* (Crown, 1988).

Melosh, Barbara. *"The Physician's Hand": Work Culture and Conflict in American Nursing.* Philadelphia: Temple University Press, 1982.
This history of nursing from the 1920s to the 1970s views that history through the lenses of work culture, the rules, customs, and behaviors associated with a particular work or workplace. Melosh treats her subject from the perspective of women's experience of the work of nursing rather than from the perspective of an analysis of the profession. The author's description of nursing as "the story of women workers' experience in a rationalizing service industry" still provides a context for reflection on that health care profession. Her conclusion describing changes in nursing at the time of the book's publication, including the impact of feminism and the future of the field, provides a lucid and helpful backdrop to the further experiences of added responsibility for nurses and further identification of them as patient advocates.

Miller, Dorothy C. *Women and Social Welfare: A Feminist Analysis.* New York: Praeger, 1990.
Miller sees that major social welfare systems in the United States exist with anachronistic rules. Proposed changes have been opposed as being antifamily. She places this reluctance to change in the fact that the social

welfare system was designed to perpetuate women's place in the nuclear family. Policy changes would impact notions of gender roles which still remain strong. This book, examining the function of gender assumptions in the social welfare system, places this examination in a feminist framework. The author's thesis is that both women's relationships to men and their status as mothers are variables which are more powerful than work ethic principles in shaping social welfare policy. She reviews feminist theories which try to explain differential treatment of gender, and she describes Aid to Families with Dependent Children (AFDC) vivis-à-visa-vis gender as well as political necessity. She pays attention to work and work training programs for poor women, noting that these perpetuate dependency and will continue to do so. Chapters 7 and 8 provide a perspective on the situation of older women in patriarchal society, most particularly through the lenses of Social Security and pensions, both of which are major considerations with regard to costs and benefits related to women and health.

Myers, Henry, ed. *Women at Work: How They're Reshaping America.* Princeton, NJ: Dow Jones Books, 1979.

Based on a series of articles originally appearing in the *Wall Street Journal* in the summer of 1978, this collection presents information on the gains and problems of women in the paid workforce by the time of its publication. Some parts are helpful history; other parts point out realities, in some respects still operative, which some might wish were history. Women at work are still shaping America and still likely to run into issues which men do not face. "Foreign Assignments" discusses working American women dealing with other cultures while working abroad. "Blue Collar and Happy" provides information on U.S. government policies with regard to companies with federal contracts having goals for hiring women in all construction craft jobs. The contemporary reader not only will find the percentages inadequate to the 1990s but also may be disheartened to hear about or to remember experiences of sex discrimination, pay inequity, and family consequences not yet resolved.

This book can be read with even greater profit in combination with *Gender Traps* by Judith Briles (McGrawHill, 1996) and *Women Workers and Global Restructuring*, edited by Kathryn Ward (ILR Press, 1990).

Norsigian, Judy. "Women and National Health Care Reform: A Progressive Feminist Agenda." In Alice J. Dan, ed., *Reframing Women's Health: Multidisciplinary Research and Practice*. Thousand Oaks, CA: Sage Publications, 1994.

Although women use the health care system more frequently than men and although women are the vast majority of health care workers, both paid and unpaid, their voices were unheard in the debate on national health care reform preceding the 1992 presidential election in the United States. In this essay, Norsigian, one of the original members of the Boston Women's Health Book Collective, collaborative authors of *Our Bodies, Ourselves*, presents the costs to women and women's health if, once again, "experts" define what women's problems are and how they ought to be solved. Being quite clear that policy makers must hear from women, Norsigian lays out the issues to which planners must attend if justice, health, and benefits concomitant to costs will function.

Payne, Elizabeth Anne. *Reform, Labor and Feminism: Margaret Drier Robins and the Women's Trade Union League*. Chicago: University of Illinois Press, 1988.

This book is not only a biography of Margaret Drier but also a history of the Women's Trade Union League. The history provides an analysis of the ideals and aspirations of the WTUL, which offered a home to reform-oriented women looking to address the implications, social and civic, of the new industrial order. Founded in 1903, the WTUL joined feminist ideals and labor reforms in its commitment to change society by addressing the problems of workers and the urban poor, with a specific orientation to organize and protect female wage earners. The diversity of

WTUL members mirrored their belief that women could gather across ethnic and class barriers to confront social injustice. The author finds that Margaret Drier Robins, president of the WTUL from 1907 to 1922, and the Women's Trade Union League illuminate in their joint stories an important aspect of early twentieth century reform and show the values of a significant branch of Progressivism.

Quaid, Maeve. *Job Evaluation: The Myth of Equitable Assessment.* New York: University of Toronto Press, 1993.
Arguing that both mainstream human resource management and feminists have misinterpreted the nature of formal job evaluation techniques, the author shows that these misinterpretations apply especially to resolving current pay equity debates. Seeing beyond the rational and political interpretations of job evaluation, Quaid considers the symbolic. She uses, as her means of critique, both institutional theory and social constructivism, leading ultimately to her definition of job evaluation as an institutionalized myth.

Raffo, Susan, ed. *Queerly Classed.* Boston: South End Press, 1997.
Exploring the intersections of social status, class background, and "queerness," this work is a collection of essays displaying reflectivity, honesty, and courage. It bypasses stereotypes, opening up narrow and/or rigid descriptions of gay and lesbian communities. The contributors, in offering essays on family, relationships, money, and home, deal with questions of privilege and poverty, pride and shame, and community and alienation. The authors point out the impact of intertwined forms of inequality on self-understanding, on empowerment, and on activism. Indirectly, this work, redefining class and "queerness," shows the larger cost to society in health care inequities, including those incurred by being family in an alternative manner, those involved in being a caretaker with no formal rights, and those hidden in the complicated and conflicting emotions clustered around invisibility.

Scott, Niki. *The Working Woman: A Handbook.* Kansas City: Universal
    Press Syndicate, 1977.
    This book offers working women a look at how other working women
    cope with their problems. It is encouraging in allowing the reader to
    understand that other women experience anger at unfair treatment in the
    workplace, are exhausted at still doing more than their share of
    housework and childrearing, or are single and without the supports that
    couples have. The publication date of this book might lead one to believe
    that its concerns and the experiences shared in it no longer exist;
    however, though the statistics have changed, a good portion of women's
    experience around these issues has not. Without a doubt, women still
    face discrimination, both personal and economic, in the workforce. The
    author, a freelance writer, was at one time a nationally syndicated
    columnist whose "Working Woman" appeared biweekly in 200
    newspapers.

Sen, Gita, Adrienne Germain, and C. Chen. *Population Policies
    Reconsidered: Health, Empowerment and Human Rights.* Cambridge,
    MA: Harvard University Press, 1994.
    A collection of articles from a diverse group of scholars, policy makers,
    and women's health activists, this work explores future directions for
    population policies with an emphasis on health, empowerment, and
    human rights.

Shiva, Vandana. *Biopiracy: The Plunder of Nature and Knowledge.*
    Boston: South End Press, 1997.
    In this clearly argued and highly principled book, the author, a physicist,
    activist, and internationally renowned Third World environmentalist,
    explores what she sees as the latest frontier of the North's rape of the
    South's biological resources. Now that land, atmosphere, forests, and
    oceans have already been colonized, she sees Northern capital as carving
    out new regions to exploit for gain: the inner recesses of women's
    bodies, plants, and animals. Shiva finds that some trade agreements

protect the North so that it is free to steal from the Third World's genetic diversity. She argues that this has serious consequences for women, for the Third World, and for the environment. The book pays specific attention to gene patenting, genetic engineering, and biotechnology. This book will have appeal for the reader concerned not only with feminism but also with the environment, technology, or colonization. It deals ultimately with costs to the exosphere as well as costs to women's health.

Smith, Patricia, ed. *Feminist Jurisprudence*. New York: Oxford University Press, 1993.

This book, in presenting its information, provides the reader an opportunity to arrive at the legal costs, both financial and personal, arising from inadequate approaches to understandings of women as full human persons and from inadequate approaches to women's whole health. It ultimately speaks to the health of the body politic and to the total costs to society of not tending to women's health. While these issues are treated indirectly, there are more direct considerations which can be mentioned. The introduction, "Feminist Jurisprudence and the Nature of Law," offers an excellent discussion of the types of feminism, presenting benefits and drawbacks of each. It is profitably read in conjunction with Rosemarie Tong's *Feminist Thought: A Comprehensive Introduction* (Westview Press, 1989). Chapter 4, "The Emergence of Feminist Jurisprudence: An Essay" by Ann C. Scales, speaks to the tyranny of objectivity, mentioning feminist method in connection with Gilligan's distinction between rights based and care based ethics. She places the reality of the question in a compulsion to control as distinct from a commitment to restrain. Reading Carol Gilligan's *In a Different Voice* (Harvard University Press, 1982) helps the reader with a context for Scales' discussion. The whole of Part II, "On Justice and Harm: Battery, Harassment, and Rape," sees these issues as illustrations of sexism and fits well with consideration of these realities as women's health issues. Chapter 12, "Reproductive Freedom," by Deborah L. Rhode, presents a helpful historical background and addresses both abortion and adolescent pregnancy. Reading Linda Gordon's *Women's Body, Women's Right* (Grossman, 1977), as well as Kristin Luker's *Abortion and the Politics of Motherhood* (University of California Press, 1984), provides further context for Rhode's discussion.

Spain, Daphne, and Suzanne M. Bianchi. *Balancing Act: Motherhood, Marriage and Employment Among American Women.* New York: Russell Sage Foundation, 1996.
Although the gap between men's and women's salaries has shrunk, and although women have made significant gains in education and in the workforce, women still hold significantly lower-paying positions and are still paid less than men. This book makes note of the fact that as women have established a greater presence outside the home, they have not only delayed marriage and motherhood but also have been left alone to balance the demands of both care giving and wage earning. As the only industrialized nation lacking policies to support working mothers and their families, the United States makes the risk of poverty the single greatest danger facing American women. Contributing to the national dialogue concerning family policy, welfare reform, and responsibility for children, this book points out, at least indirectly, the possible consequences of health care reform on women's poverty and women's health. As the health care system calls upon women to continue to do more with less, the cost not only to women but also to the nation as a whole can be devastating.

Statham, Anne, Eleanor Miller, and Hans O. Mauksch, eds. *The Worth of Women's Work: A Qualitative Analysis.* Albany: State University of New York Press, 1987.
This collection of essays on women and work includes an exploration of women's work roles, both paid and unpaid, including teachers, nurses, social workers, domestic workers, factory workers, and managers. It considers women's approaches to work as well as specific kinds of work and correlative policy. The editors are of the opinion, which they express

in "The Qualitative Approach to the Study of Women's Work: Different Method/Different Knowledge," that qualitative approaches to data gathering put the accent on the perspective of those being studied. Such approaches view those studied as actively constructing their own experience. This is quite different from assuming the rightness of the dominant view and proceeding accordingly. Clearly, qualitative approaches, which are the editors' preference, are more appropriate to a wider interpretation of costs and benefits.

Tomaskovic-Devy, Donald, ed. *Poverty and Social Welfare in the United States*. Boulder, CO: Westview Press, 1988.
In his introductory essay, the editor of this collection provides a broad overview and a roadmap for the reader. He shows that poverty is damaging to the individual and, by extension, to the society, since money and goods are key to social participation. He points out that the two best predictors of official poverty status in the United States are sex and race. He names hiring discrimination and structural barriers to labor force participation as accounting for part of the higher rates of poverty among blacks and females. The chapters most pertinent for consideration in this annotated bibliography are Chapter 2, "The Feminization of Poverty: Nature, Causes, and a Partial Cure," Chapter 3, "Unmarried Women in a Patriarchal Society: Impoverishment and Access to Health Care Across the Life-Cycle," Chapter 7, "Fighting Poverty by Reducing Dependency: The Dilemma of Policy Assumptions," and Chapter 9, "Health and Poverty in Single-Parent Families: The Consequences of Federal Policy Change." These essays show female poverty in a patriarchal society as directly reflective of its traditional subordination of women.

Ward, Kathryn, ed. *Women Workers and Global Restructuring*. Ithaca, NY: ILR Press, Cornell University, 1990.
This volume presents some of the more recent research on women, work, and the restructuring of the global economy. The editor notes that in the developing countries, this restructuring is shown in the growth of the

service sector and in the specialization in export industries. She finds that the growth in the informal sector and women workers is the centerpiece of this restructuring. Recent research has also explored the links between global restructuring and housework, informal sector work, and formal labor. Women in many parts of the world, including the United States, now work triple shifts: housework, homework, and formal waged work. Where researchers once focused on class, gender, and race as additive factors, they now examine the interrelated effects of these as primary issues. Informal sector work is the intermediate link between formal waged labor and housework. It is unprotected waged labor, which, when performed by women in the home, without pay and without Social Security, is called housework. The contributors to this book touch on themes of redefining work, juggling formal and informal labor, and housework. They consider the costs and benefits of transnational corporation employment. They discuss the intersections of race, gender, and class. They employ a variety of research methods. They focus on nations at the core, the semiperiphery, and the periphery of the global economy. In terms of the costs and benefits connected with women and health, one might ask if "Doctor Mom," or women who are called upon to do for loved ones what health care system services used to do, are part of the growth in the informal sector. Will informal sector work be the centerpiece of United States health care reform?

Weiner, Lynn Y. *From Working Girl to Working Mother: The Female Labor Force in the United States, 1820-1980.* Chapel Hill: University of North Carolina Press, 1985.

In this history of women and work in the United States, Weiner moves from the development of the idea of the "working girl" to more contemporary controversies over working mothers. Presenting two clearly distinguishable phases in the progression of women's labor, 1820 to 1920, and 1920 to the publication of this book, the author shows the changes in the lives of working women reflected in the female work force's transition from single, female, self-supporting workers to the predominance of married women and mothers. Her chapters deal with attitudes toward women and work as well as relationships between women and the social order, through discussing such topics as immigration, working women's associations, and ideas of motherhood and family. In seeing the larger pipicture, Weiner concludes that improved child care and changed notions of work will benefit the whole of society, not only working women. In its tables and bibliography, this work provides help for the reader.

Wimberly, Anne Streaty, ed. *Honoring African American Elders: A Ministry in the Soul Community*. San Francisco: Jossey-Bass, 1997.
Considering the fact that older adults are the fastest growing segment not only of the population of the United States in general but also of the African American population of churchgoers in particular, the author explores the church's role for these elders. She expresses the importance of preparing church leaders for responding effectively to the needs of this segment of congregations. Offering a paradigm for a ministry which restores African American elders to their place of importance, she proposes concrete ways for making this ministry a viable reality, both for the elders and for the whole community of which they are part. Although this book directly addresses pastoral care for African American elders, it is a valuable resource for all who work with senior members of any church congregation.

Wright, Barbara Drygulski, Myra Marx Ferret, Gail O. Mellow, Linda H. Lewis, Maria Luz Daza Samper, Robert Asher, and Kathleen Claspell, eds. *Women, Work, and Technology: Transformations*. Ann Arbor: University of Michigan Press, 1987.
Recognizing that technology has to deal with the social environment and the responses of nonexperts, the introduction, written by Barbara Wright, rejects the concept that humans are technologically determined, that is, limited in their responses to technology. This book is an interdisciplinary collection comprising essays and research considering the impact on

women of workplace technology. The essays include historical discussions as well as contemporary issues. Among these are reproductive health and safety issues vis-à-vis new technology, changes in the dynamics of work, and the influence of computers. Computer equity for women, flight attendants' unions, and technology's impact upon farm workers are also addressed in these essays.

ADDICTIONS

INTRODUCTION

The last decades of the twentieth century have seen a new clarity in dealing with addictions. Although the word itself was first associated with alcoholism, as far as data and understanding were concerned, it moved through other research. Until the 1980s women were still seen to be less involved with alcohol and/or other drugs. Part of that view was intimately connected to cultural descriptions of women as well as moral descriptions of addiction.

With the advent of the "disease" concept of alcoholism, through the 1945 survey of Dr. Jellinek and later through the American Medical Assoication's naming of alcoholism as a disease, came the understanding of addiction as a health issue rather than a moral one. As information about addictions other than alcoholism grew, treatment became an industry. As Dr. Jane E. James, in 1975, picked up on the questionnaires filled out by women but left out of Jellinek's 1945 survey, concern about women's experience and particular needs in treatment of alcoholism grew. Even though, as with other diseases, women were left out of the research subjects until closer to the 1990s, knowledge of their experiences, concerns, and needs was a concern among clusters of health care providers, particularly treatment personnel.

Holistic concerns with regard to health have increased as mind-body connections have become clearer. It was quite natural then that addictions, having been seen as diseases involving mind, body, and spirit, would attract more attention in the general public. More and more women came out of the hiddenness and silence of their addictions. More and more, they began to receive some of the help needed.

The entries in this section deal with women and addiction as part of women's whole health across the lifespan. They concern not only information about women and addictions but also considerations on larger societal issues. They also pay attention to how treatment language has helped and sometimes hurt women in their quest for wholeness around addictions issues. In this section, care of women and care by women are conflated.

While theological and religious works were included primarily in the first section of this bibliography, "Descriptions of Women," spirituality books will be included in this one. Though one cannot so easily distinguish between the two in terms of theoretical and practical focus, or intellectual and affective, suffice it to say that spirituality, as a way of seeing and of being in the world, is a crucial factor in the recovery process and in the healing process. This is the primary reason I have included it in this chapter. Spirituality becomes particularly worthy of attention as a tool of honesty, sobriety, freedom, and wholeness, all of which are issues pertinent to addiction and recovery.

Even in addictions health the interconnections between social constructs of women and gender and their relationship to diagnostic terminology hold true. A prime example is the psychiatric pathology for masochistic personality disorders in the DSM-III-R, *Diagnostic and Statistical Manual of Mental Disorders*, third edition (American Psychiatric Association, 1987). It was listed as the syndrome "self-defeating personality disorder," and placed in the Appendix, that is, those issues needing further research and not yet to be used as diagnoses. The custom is to give such listings no code number by which they may be referred to as diagnoses and entered for third-party payment. In fact "self-defeating personality disorder" and what people commonly call "PMS" (premenstrual syndrome), although placed in the appendix, were given code numbers, unlike any listings before or since. The kind of issues called self-defeating behaviors are actually culturally approved, if not prescribed, ways for women to behave. Making this note hardly attends to the fact that the behaviors mentioned may be good coping strategies for battered women, some of whom are killed when they break free. In addiction and recovery concerns, sometimes the language of codependency is used in such a way that it pathologizes women for using societally recommended behaviors. As for premenstrual syndrome, which was ultimately provided another name and approved into the text of the DSM IV, *Diagnostic and Statistical Manual of Mental Disorders*, fourth edition, it represents a pathology based upon female hormone fluctuation. There is no similar pathology for men based upon their hormonal situation.

ANNOTATIONS

Allen, Paula Gunn. *Grandmothers of the Light: A Medicine Woman's Sourcebook*. Boston: Beacon Press, 1991.
   Paula Gunn Allen, herself part Native American, presents myths and stories from a range of Native American peoples: Aztec, Cherokee, Iroquois, Navaho, and Pueblo. Showing that "myth" and "mother," though discredited in a modern world, are nonetheless essential to the world's existence, Allen shows myth as medicine stories, stories of sacred power. Her first section is a cosmogony, a universe in harmony with gynocratic, or female ruling principles, some of which are egalitarianism, personal autonomy, communal harmony, and complementarity. The myths, as Gunn understands them in this first section, show a spiritual system in harmony with gynocentric values of peace, tolerance, sharing, balance, and harmony. For women working at recovery in androcentric societies, this first section is not only delightful but also empowering. Both the introduction, "The Living Reality of the Medicine World," and the postscript supply a context for this three-sectioned book

Anderson, Peggy K. *Coming Home: Adult Children of Alcoholics*. Seattle, WA: Glen Abbey Books, 1988.
   In relating the story of two young children whose father is in alcohol treatment, this book points out issues such as the children's loss of trust in family relations and difficulties with studies and friendships. The work

is intended to encourage the healing of adult children of alcoholics with regard to the feelings and experiences they underwent being raised in an alcoholic surrounding. Given its large print, illustrations, and text, it is also helpful and appropriate for children. At the end of the work there is a "child's page," encouraging children to share feelings and anxieties concerning a parent's alcoholism with a trusted adult, such as a friend, relative, or teacher. Included are a list of organizations and resources for reading for adult children of alcoholics.

Anderson, Sherry Ruth, and Patricia Hopkins. *The Feminine Face of God: The Unfolding of the Sacred in Women.* New York: Bantam, 1991.

This work provides a space within which women can see themselves and their own spirituality. In interviewing women from varying backgrounds - poet Maya Angelou, women in a spiritual community, a rabbi, a former nun, and a Seneca elder - the authors present a range of experiences of spirituality. The diverse backgrounds and viewpoints presented point out an ongoing need and an ongoing benefit in sharing the unfolding of the sacred in women across life and spirituality contexts.

Beattie, Melody. *Beyond Codependency.* New York: Harper and Row, 1989.

This book builds upon the author's previous publication, *Codependent No More* (Harper/Hazelden, 1987), in addressing those who are recovering from issues of chemical dependency, or codependency or are adult children of alcoholics. Whereas *Codependent No More* dealt with stopping pain and gaining control of life, this book discusses continuing growing after the pain has stopped. *Codependent No More* was a call and a set of information and advice about beginning recovery; this book is about working on the issues of recovery, about a honing of skills. Comprising five sections plus an epilogue and a bibliography, the book addresses such issues as the process of recovery, breaking through shame, boundaries, intimacy, and sharing recovery with one's children.

Beattie opens each chapter with a pertinent quote and closes with practical activities. This is not simply a reading book; it is also a doing book. Chapter 16, on intimacy, is well read in conjunction with Janet Woititz's *Struggle for Intimacy* (Health Communications, 1985).

Beattie, Melody. *The Language of Letting Go.* Center City, MN: Hazelden, 1990.
This book of meditations encourages the reader to spend some daily time in the process of reflection, many times remembering what she already knows. While it is written primarily for the self-care of women in recovery, particularly those who see themselves as recovering from codependency, it is suitable for all women attempting to find meaning and enhance quality in their lives. Ordinary experiences and questions, such as those pertaining to dealing with grief, finding direction, enhancing honesty in relationships, knowing boundaries, accepting feelings, and owning one's own energy are among the topics addressed in the 365 meditations offered. One of the beauties of this book is its ability to supply brief, pointed reflections which can be recollected and built upon during the day. Each meditation ends with a combination affirmation/prayer/resolution.

Bepko, Claudia, with JoAnn Krestan. *The Responsibility Trap: A Blueprint for Treating the Alcoholic Family.* New York: The Free Press, 1985.
Examining the dynamics of families with the particular dysfunction of alcoholism, the authors use a family systems method. They analyze behaviors and patterns within the family and consider the transmission of alcoholic behavior over generations. They then provide guidelines for intervention and treatment. In a separate chapter, they discuss children of alcoholics and the treatment process. Considering survival roles adopted by the children, they highlight the problems of adjustment after the alcoholic parent arrives at sobriety. In a brief section on adult children of alcoholics, the authors provide specific treatment goals which

are based in personal experience. Well grounded in family theory and practical experience concerning alcoholism counseling, this book, intended for professionals, may be profitably read by alcoholics and family members.

Berger, Louis S. *Substance Abuse as Symptom*. Hillsdale, NJ: The Analytic Press, 1991.

Showing that the psychoanalytic tradition has long been interested in substance abuse, Berger points out that compulsive drug use has been seen in that tradition as a symptom of severe pathology. Thus, patients with drug addiction problems are generally identified as having severe personality disorders. Examining whether there are other ways in which a psychoanalytic framework can make a contribution, the author applies the psychoanalytic framework, first at the cultural level, then at the clinical level. In working from these levels he sees that there is a pervasive and severe cultural psychopathology which accounts for a number of aspects of the substance abuse problem. Thus, he sets out to examine the drug problem in that wider context of sociocultural symptoms and problems. He draws upon analytic thought and clinical wisdom for this. His reconceptualizing of substance abuse within a wider sociocultural context in Part I is followed by clinical concerns in Part II. What is most helpful to the non-professional person reading this work is the author's articulation of widely accepted ideas as to what substance abuse is, how it might be prevented, and how it ought to be treated. The reader, either professional or non-professional, having followed Berger's information and arguments, can then sift the fittingness of his conclusions.

Berry, Carmen Renee. *When Helping You Is Hurting Me*. San Francisco: Harper and Row, 1988.

A combination of the author's professional experience and her personal growth experience, this book addresses helping persons who fall into what Berry calls the "messiah trap," a situation she describes in her first chapter. The book continues in the direction of naming the trap, even where it is hidden, considering characteristics and types of "messiahs," and laying out advice and strategies for avoiding or coming out of that trap. Appendix A, "How to Find the Help You Need," provides opportunities for assistance, and modes of selection among those opportunities. Appendix B, "The Victim-Offender-Messiah Response Pattern to the Victimization Experience" provides a schema, a sense of trends in the literature, and a listing of treatment issues for persons in that triad. While the reader may not have concretely experienced the victim or offender situation which elicited this book, the insights concerning loving oneself as one helps others is pertinent for the reader's general well-being.

Buonaventura, Wendy. *Serpent of the Nile: Women and Dance in the Arab World.* Brooklyn, NY: Interlink Books, 1990.
Buonaventura presents the development of Arabic dance as an art and as a profession. She highlights the fact that, unlike some forms of entertainment, belly dancing and other forms of Arabic dance do not require the professional performer to be young or slender. Surviving hundreds of years until the twentieth century, Arabic dance became a Westernized entertainment. Buonaventura, herself a performer of the dance of which she speaks, points out the antiquity of the use of dance and its identification of fertility with a mother goddess. The sense of mythology, the cultural contribution, and the sense of comfort about the female body make this work useful for recovering women.

Carlson, Karen J., M.D., Stephanie A. Eisenstadt, M.D., and Terra Ziporyn, Ph.D. *The Harvard Guide to Women's Health.* Cambridge, MA: Harvard University Press, 1996.
The entries on addictions in this guide are listed under specific dependencies: alcohol, caffeine, smoking, and substance abuse. The beauty of the considerations on each is that they are interwoven with the

related health problems beyond each specific addiction. These are listed in the "related entries" at the end of each entry as well as in the subject index. The section on alcohol addiction presents symptoms along with practical self-questions and modes of treatment. The discussion on caffeine lists its effects as well as providing a set of tables showing caffeine amounts in substances most commonly used by ordinary women. It links coffee with possibly related diseases. The entry on smoking lists the effects of that habit on the respiratory system, on the cardiovascular system, on the reproductive system, on the musculoskeletal system, on the skin, and on the health of other family members. It discusses the benefits of quitting and helpful ways of accomplishing it. The entry on substance abuse deals with both illegal and prescription drugs, including symptoms and treatment, presenting helpful charts listing types of drugs, symptoms of overuse or abuse, and common symptoms of withdrawal.

Casey, Karen. *Each Day a New Beginning.* Center City, MN: Hazelden, 1982.

One of the early women's recovery meditation books, this work is printed by Hazelden, a major treatment center as well as a research and publications house. The author, who originally chose to be anonymous, gives back what she has received from women "as sisters, as equal travelers on our parallel spiritual journeys." She has learned to hear women and in turn gives them voice by beginning each day's reflective meditation with a quotation from a woman. Her quotations include women whose names are immediately recognizable as well as women who are extraordinary by being ordinary. While some readers may find individual meditations neither to their liking nor consistent with their current belief system, there is still something for all in this book. Though it is not annotated in this volume, a companion book, *The Promise of a New Day,* by Karen Casey and Martha Vanceburg (Hazelden, 1983) is also a book of daily meditations. It is not, however, written only for women.

Casey, Karen. *If Only I Could Quit: Becoming a Non-Smoker.* San Francisco: Harper and Row, 1987.

This book encourages a smoke-free existence by presenting stories told to Casey by "recovering" smokers willing to share their experiences, their hope, and their courage. This invitation and encouragement by those who have gone before provides the reader with motivation as well as strategies folded into the stories of the quitters. Because of the range of situations and experiences represented (gender, social status, age, profession) most readers are able to find points of identification with some or other of the storytellers. This recognition tends to open insight, bringing readers back to themselves and their unique situation and needs. The book also presents 90 daily meditations, since most people find the first three months free of nicotine the most difficult. The quotations preceding each meditation are words spoken by the storytellers during their interviews. The author encourages each reader to accept the support given by the meditations and to return to the first meditation if, after 90 days, he or she is not so comfortable a nonsmoker as might be desired.

Cavanaugh, Eunice, M.Ed., M.S.W. *Understanding Shame: Why It Hurts, How It Helps, How You Can Use It to Transform Your Life.* Minneapolis, MN: Johnson Institute, 1989.

This book serves this annotated bibliography in two ways. It is published by the Johnson Institute, a research and treatment center for addictions and the family, and it deals with shame, a key element both in addiction and in recovery. In the introduction, Cavanaugh places shame as the antithesis of love. Then she divides her work into three parts: "Shame, Guilt, Anger, and the Self," "The Shame-Anxiety Cycle," and "Overcoming Barriers to Change." Her afterward, "The Courage to Heal," is an encouragement which shares the poem of a woman healing. The author provides a listing of "Mutual Help and Networking Groups" and a bibliography, "For Further Reading." One beauty of this book is that it deals with what has been perceived as a negative subject in a positive way: Cavanaugh discusses the value of shame and anger.

Another help is the author's diagrams, which are clear, concisely laying out both a scope and a review. Her picture of the shame-anxiety cycle (p. 38), for example, points toward the material following and later can serve the reader as a memory tool.

Chollat-Tranquet, C. *Women and Tobacco*. Geneva: World Health Organization, 1992.
A global overview of current trends in female smoking. Produced with the support of WHO, this book highlights the growing number of women smokers around the world and documents the likely health effects.

Cousins, Norman. *Head First: The Biology of Hope and the Healing Power of the Human Spirit*. New York: Penguin Books, 1989.
Although this book has some medical flavor and ultimately deals with psychoneuroimmunology, the practicality of its approach becomes a fine self-education to recovery and the human spirit. Particularly helpful in terms of recovery from addictions, not directly but rather by implication, are Chapter 5, "The Infinite Wonder of the Human Brain," Chapter 9, "Problems Beyond the Doctor's Reach," Chapter 10, "The Laughter Connection," Chapter 12, "Mesmer, Hypnotism, and the Powers of the Mind," and Chapter 13, "Firewalking." The reader who enjoys this book will quite likely be interested in another of Cousins' works, *The Healing Heart* (Avon Books, 1983).

Craighead, Meinrad. *The Litany of the Great River*. New York: Paulist Press, 1991.
Each with a text for reflection and one of the author's paintings, the litanies in this book praise the earth. Craighead is a former nun who belonged to a contemplative order and is an artist surrounded by the earth tones of New Mexico. Steeped in traditional Catholic culture and informed by Native American spirituality and women's wisdom, Craighead, without necessarily intending to, offers women in recovery a spiritual depth inviting them back to their own bodies and to a flow of

life. Her art, in earth tones, featuring women who seem formed from the earth, is a wonderful corrective to spiritualities which have perceived earth and body, represented by woman, as evil or lesser.

Craighead, Meinrad. *The Mother's Songs: Images of God the Mother.* Mahwah, NJ: Paulist Press, 1986.

Comprising seventy-nine of the artist's renditions, with her corresponding meditations, this book is a powerful statement and a powerful encouragement for women's spirit. The names and images of God the Mother not only are reminiscent of the goddess/creatrix myths of other religions and cultures, but also are clearly part of the Catholic religion and culture. Some names and images are hidden, some only pointed toward, some actually named in the *Litany of the Blessed Virgin Mary.* Craighead, artist and author, comes from a grandmother and a mother whose spirits remain present to her. Her imagery begins in the "pulse beat" she learned from her grandmother's body as her grandmother, a storyteller, gave voice to her imagination. As Craighead draws from her deep source, her art and meditation encourage the same in her readers and her viewers.

David, Jay, ed. *The Family Secret: An Anthology.* New York: William Morrow and Company, 1994.

Presented in four parts, this book moves beyond the broader truths concerning alcoholism, as well as the generalizations and the statistics. The editor, aware that every story is unique, gathers the stories of successful and well-known people who have survived childhood in an alcoholic family and who have shown a resiliency and triumph of spirit. This book intends to be, and is, a sign of hope. While the stories, in fact, surpass the broader truths about alcoholism, the editor uses some of those truths as his four divisions: that families hide the disease, that often the children are abused, that alcoholic parents tend to die early, and that children of alcoholics tend to abuse alcohol. These truths are expressed in "The Family Secret," "Living in Fear," "Early Exit," and "It Runs in the Family."

Duerk, Judith. *Circle of Stones: Women's Journey to Herself.* San Diego: Lura Media, 1991.

Presenting "what if" kinds of questions, Duerk illuminates a healing journey fueled by a re-listening to the ancient voice of the feminine. Employing and inviting a retreat mode, the author encourages envisioning a world where women can retire to women's space and, finding the guidance of their elders, discover new balance. In three sections-"In Search of Her Mother," "In Search of Her Self," and "In Search of Her Life"-the book models, by its existence and by its dynamic, the unfolding of a woman's dream. The work intertwines dreams, images, and experiences with sufficient contextualizing information to encourage the reader to do reflective exercises beneficial to herself and to the fostering of her own dreams and images. Each reflective piece begins with, "How might your life have been different if. . ." and ends with "How might your life be different?" The tapestries woven among past, present, and future foster this weaving within and across women.

Dulfano, Celia. *Families, Alcoholism, and Recovery.* San Francisco: Jossey-Bass, 1992.

In this revised edition, Dulfano, a pioneer in studying the impact of alcoholism on the family, updates and expands her work, offering additional case studies and maturing concepts of the family systems model for therapeutic intervention. This is particularly helpful in a treatment field which has a relatively recent history. This book can be used not only by professionals but also by any family member related to an active or a recovering alcoholic. The author uses inclusive language by alternating masculine and feminine pronouns, in an attempt to avoid sexism. Part I stresses the value of family treatment, discussing the necessity for expanding treatments and recognizing the legitimacy of focusing on family offspring. Part II employs case studies highlighting typical issues which arise in treatment, for example individual sobriety without the treatment of family patterns, mechanisms of denial in the alcoholic, family collusion in hiding problems, and problems particular to low-income families. Part III, "Women, Family Therapy, and Alcoholism," is most pertinent to this annotated bibliography. Chapter 13 in this division affords the reader an example of multimodal psychotherapy in its application to a group of daughters and wives of alcoholics. These women were treated in a combined group therapy and family therapy modality, with useful results. In summarizing various therapeutic techniques, Chapter 14 points to the requisites of tailoring family therapy to alcoholism.

Fields, Richard, Ph.D. *Drugs in Perspective.* Madison, WI: Brown and Benchmark, 1995.

With its major emphasis on family dynamics, this second edition of *Drugs in Perspective* is different from the traditional pharmacological text. Its eleven chapters aim at offering readers an understanding of the general dynamics of chemical dependency and an encouragement to come to their own perspectives on dependence and addiction. The book is extremely practical, containing easily understood tables and illustrations, case studies, common questions most readers might have, and chapter summaries. Some chapters contain worksheets assisting readers to formulate their own perspectives. Because its major emphasis is on family dynamics, the book contextualizes its considerations on alcohol and other drugs within an individual's family system and shows the devastating toll on family members as well as the benefits in recovery. Chapter 3, in its outlining of a behavioral definition of addiction, presents the author's perspectives and invites readers to establish theirs. Chapter 5 treats the feelings in dysfunctional family systems, particularly the impact of shame. Chapter 7, the newly developed chapter in this second edition, treats depressive disorders and personality disorders, issues sometimes overlooked in textbooks concerning alcohol and other drugs. One particularly helpful aspect of this book is its clear and manageable layout. This book is a good companion to Sharon Wegschieder's *Another Chance* (Science and Behavior Books, 1981) and Eunice Cavanaugh's *Understanding Shame* (Johnson Institute, 1989).

Frances, Richard J., M.D., and John E. Franklin, M.D. *A Concise Guide to Treatment of Alcoholism and Addictions.* Washington, DC: American Psychiatric Press, 1989.

Addressing topics of great concern to psychiatrists, the Concise Guide series contains pocket-sized compendia of brief but relevant information. This volume emphasizes treatment issues. It discusses the magnitude of the problem, economic costs, medical and psychiatric concerns, and complications of denial. Summarizing developmental issues in the field, the authors provide considerations on the evolution of the disease concept of alcoholism and an emphasis on more recent trends toward prevention. They discuss diagnosis, alluding to the DSM-III-R and the DSM-IV and considering the criteria used to diagnose substance dependence and abuse. For the purposes of this annotated bibliography, the section on special populations is most relevant. While women are afforded approximately three pages, those pages are helpful, not only for what they say but also for what they model in terms of assumptions.

Graham, Kathryn, Sarah J. Saunders, Margaret C. Flower, Carol Birchmore Timney, Marilyn White-Campbell, and Anne Zeidman Pietropaolo. *Addiction Treatment for Older Adults: Evaluation of an Innovative Client-Centered Approach.* New York: The Haworth Press, 1995.

For gerontologists, epidemiologists, and clinicians working with older adults experiencing problems related to the use of alcohol and/or other drugs, this book is also for anyone who is interested. It discusses the results of evaluative research at the COPA (Community Older Persons Alcohol) program. The program's philosophy differs from other addictions treatment programs in that there is no requirement for clients to admit they have a problem in order to receive help and each person is allowed to determine her/his own treatment needs. Chapters 1 and 2 provide a description of the program and its rationale. Perhaps most helpful for the reader who is neither a clinician nor a researcher in the field are Chapter 3, "A Topology of COPA Clients," Chapter 5, "Literature Review of the Factors Relating to Drinking Problems Among Older Adults," Chapter 7, "Problems of Older Alcohol and Drug Abusers," and Chapter 11, "Conclusions." Both appendices-"Client Contact Record" and, "LESA Assessment Form,"-are helpful to professionals and nonprofessionals alike. This program combines the innovative and the successful.

Greenleaf, Jael. *Co-Alcoholic, Para-Alcoholic: Who's Who and What's the Difference.* Denver: MAC Publishing, 1981.

One of the earlier considerations on the dysfunctions and needs of those related to alcoholics and suffering from the dynamics of the disease process of the addiction as well as their responses to it, this booklet makes a distinction between the spouse of the addicted person and the children of the same. Greenleaf describes the co-alcoholic as the spouse, or other adult partner, who helps to maintain some social and financial balance for the family. This individual's help is necessary for the alcoholic to continue in functioning. Greenleaf describes para-alcoholics as the children growing up in the alcoholic family, whose behaviors are patterned on the unhealthy roles of the parents. The work places more emphasis upon para-alcoholics and the problems they tend to develop. Greenleaf names three causes of depression in COAs and points out some of their common behaviors, such as denial and perfectionism. This work also outlines barriers to effective treatment for children of alcoholics and calls for development of programs which focus on the specific, and different, needs of spouses and children.

Guide to Clinical Preventive Services, second edition. Report of the U.S. Preventive Services Task Force. Baltimore: Williams and Wilkins, 1996.

Chapter 52, "Screening for Problem Drinking" points out the growing recognition that diagnosed alcoholism represents only one end of the spectrum of "problem drinking." Problem or heavy drinkers without typical signs of alcohol dependence are more common among patients seen in the primary care setting. Nondependent heavy drinkers, however, account for most of the alcohol-related morbidity and mortality in the general population. This chapter discusses alcohol use during pregnancy, the accuracy of screening tests, and the effectiveness of early detection. It considers clinical intervention, in particular the AUDIT Structured Interview. Chapter 53 deals with "Screening for Drug Abuse," and Chapter 54 treats "Counseling to Prevent Tobacco Use." While this guide is written for professionals, it is helpful to non-professionals. The references at the end of each chapter can be pursued for further learning.

Harrison, Larry, ed.   *Alcohol Problems in the Community*.   London: Routledge, 1996.
This work, based on studies in the United Kingdom, serves well in its considerations of the broader community. Noting that a disproportionate number of people who are at risk as problem drinkers will present themselves to the primary health care system and to the social work and probation systems, the author notes these persons are rarely identified as problem drinkers. Rather, those who reach alcoholism specialists are those more likely to have severe problems, that is, to be at an extreme end of the continuum. He also considers that many judged to be alcohol dependent will return to controlled or asymptomatic drinking, in contrast to the widely held view that alcoholism is a progressive and irreversible disease. He presents the case that there is a continuity of normal/abnormal behavior, both with regard to general mental health and with regard to addiction. He finds that persons with more common mental health issues and alcohol-related disabilities will resolve their issues without formal interventions. This book was written primarily to address the connections between social factors (poverty, homelessness, racism, and gender-based discrimination), and the incidence and prevalence of

drinking problems. It seeks to explore the implications of these relationships for mainstream community services. The essays deal with such topics as intergenerational links, youth, older people, people with learning difficulties, gender divisions, and, services for women. Essays 7 and 8 are most pertinent for this annotated bibliography.

Hoffman, Eileen, M.D. "Dependent No More: Staying Strong and Addiction Free." In *Our Health, Our Lives*. New York: Bantam Books, 1995.

In this seventeenth chapter of her book, Hoffman deals with smoking, alcohol, and other drug dependency. Of particular benefit to the reader is her sifting through the meaning of codependency, so that the word not only becomes clearer but also moves away from the blaming of women for their societal roles. Hoffman links the phenomenon to social experiences which can rob women of self-esteem, at the same time that she treats the experience seriously. Paying attention to prescription drugs, Hoffman makes her reader aware of the incidence, danger, and beliefs around their usage. The author's charts and reviews are concise and practical. Of particular interest is her listing of the gender differences in alcohol abuse. This chapter is well read along with Chapter 16, "The Eating Problem: Body Image Versus Healthy Weight." The author's considerations on health and nutrition are an excellent balance and context for discussing both anorexia and bulimia.

Ketcham, Katherine, and Ginny L. Gustafson. *Living on the Edge: A Guide to Intervention for Families with Drug and Alcohol Problems*. New York: Bantam Books, 1989.

Families can coordinate their concern about a member's addiction and help to motivate the person for treatment. This book describes that process of intervention, educating the reader about the stages of addiction and the warning signs. It provides case studies from families who, recognizing the problem, participated in interventions. The book provides suggestions pertaining to preparation for intervention and the choice of a counselor/facilitator. This text can be read by older teenagers, adults, and family counselors. A helpful appendix offers basic information concerning commonly used drugs, as well as alcohol. The authors also provide a resource list of organizations and a bibliography for further information.

King, Pat. *Help for Women with Too Much to Do.* Liguori, MO: Liguori Publications, 1988.

This book presents a combination of practical advice and Christian spirituality. Written by a mother of ten children who is also an author and speaker, the book is intended for the overtired and overextended woman. It discusses the reasons for fatigue and supplies approaches to solutions for being spread too thin by life's situations. Chapter 8, "Sixteen Ways to Say No," is a pointed, clear, and concrete list of no-saying which is almost a script for those who need practice in this skill. The combination of nutritional advice and general lifestyle questions stimulates the reader's reflection. The chatty style of the book and the author's sharing of her personal experience not only help the reader to connect with the issues but also show how ordinary and widespread are the concerns of which King speaks.

Kirkpatrick, Jean, Ph.D. *Goodbye Hangovers, Hello Life: Self-Help for Women.* New York: Atheneum, 1986.

This book eventuates from the author's personal experience and from the fact that a small percentage of women alcoholics in the United States were receiving the help they needed and that those receiving help were not having the specific needs of women met. Lack of finances, lack of specifically women's treatment, the double standard, and a double secrecy for women all have played a part in these phenomena. Noting that self-help is the most effective answer over the long haul, Kirkpatrick mentions some of the special problems with which women alcoholics deal. A high percentage have known sexual abuse and molestation. A number are dually addicted, their second addiction often coming from the family physician. Most pressing, according to this author, is the alcoholic woman's lack of positive feelings for herself. The book is presented in three parts: "Drinking," "Sobriety," and "Recovery." It supplies an appendix which includes a side by side printing of the 12 Steps of Alcoholics Anonymous (AA) and the 13 Steps of Women For Sobriety (WFS). Kirkpatrick is the founder of Women For Sobriety, the first national alcoholism recovery program exclusively for women. The comparison of the 12 Steps and the 13 Steps gives the reader a clear sense of how groups of women have been able to meet their needs and support one another. At the time of this book's publication there were 200 chapters of WFS in the United States, and the program had spread to Australia, Europe, and South America.

Klein, Anne Carolyn. *Meeting the Great Bliss Queen: Buddhists, Feminists, and the Art of the Self.* Boston: Beacon Press, 1995.
Highlighting parallels between Buddhist and feminist concepts of the self, this book sets about showing how each tradition may resource the other. Using the Great Bliss Queen, an important Buddhist enlightenment symbol, as a unifying thread, Klein considers the Buddhist practice of mindfulness, a combination of serene centering and keen awareness of change, as a helpful resource for Western women. She presents compassion, which knows the self as both powerful and interdependent, as another helpful resource. In turn, she expresses feminism's ability to expand the horizons of Buddhism to encompass social, historical, and psychological questions. The author's experience of being a professor of religious studies in the United States and her three years of field work in India, Nepal, and Tibet bring a context and flow which makes the book enjoyable to read. That same context and flow encourages the reader to ask major questions concerning self , society, and religion.

Lerner, Rokelle. *Daily Affirmations for Adult Children of Alcoholics.* Pompano Beach, FL: Health Communications, 1985.

This book of reflections is intended for adults who choose to replace self-critical inner dialogue with more positive messages. It presents daily affirmations, positive, powerful, and proactive statements helping to create desired ways of thinking, feeling, and behaving. Each day's meditation reminds the reader of choice, of conscious awareness, and of ongoing change. Each entry invites not only reflection upon the affirmation and its implications but also the development of specific strategies for incorporating the affirmation into the practicalities of daily life. The beauty of this little book is that the reader takes it in daily, small, digestible pieces, but in her own experience turns it into large, personal attitudes and behaviors.

McFague, Sallie.   *Super, Natural Christians: How We Should Love Nature*. Minneapolis, MN: Fortress Press, 1997.
In this book McFague provides a reorientation for religious perspectives, from supernatural to super, natural. She asks the reader to see the earth as Christians have been taught and exhorted to see human persons, that is, as made in the *imago dei*, the image of God. She draws the implications of such thoughts and vision by considering such topics as city planning, photography, hiking, and gardening. She also discusses incarnation, embodiments, and sacramentality. The tone and concepts of this work provide women in recovery a combination of thought, affect, and respect for body and earth which can encourage the integration and grounding essential for that recovery.

Miller, Norman S., ed.   *The Principles and Practice of Addictions in Psychiatry*. Philadelphia, PA: W. B. Saunders, 1997.
While, in terms of percentage, this collection of essays has no appreciable amount of information and concern regarding the specificity of women and addictions, it does discuss treatment for childbearing and for pregnant persons. The book is useful to readers who would like to gather what it does have. The title and existence of this book point to the

fact that addictions issues have taken a central importance in the field of psychiatry. Since more than 50% of psychiatric patients have substance abuse disorders, the *Diagnostic and Statistical Manual*, both *III* and *IV*, has given addiction a relatively independent status. The trend toward primary care medicine will likely mean addictions treatment at that level, and paid for by health care maintenance organizations. Ongoing advances in clinical research and skills have developed a broad base of practice. This work, then, is written for professionals, though it can be read with profit by interested nonprofessionals. It witnesses the reality of a specialization in addiction psychiatry and addiction medicine with board certification requirements and fellowships in the field. The approach of the book is given in its divisions: "Etiology," "Neurobiology," "Diagnosis," "Treatment Approach," "Treatment Process," and "Pharmacological Treatments." The sections on treatment approach and process are of greatest interest to the nonprofessional.

National Institute on Alcohol Abuse and Alcoholism. *Services for Alcoholic Women: Foundations for Change*. DHEW Publication No. (ADM) 79-873. Washington, DC: Government Printing Office, 1979. This resource book provides selected articles pertinent for understanding the differences in treatment needs where women are concerned. It also provides course materials for professional addictions personnel. It considers special populations of women, such as Mexican American women and lesbian women. Section III, "Treatment Program Resources," deals with collecting and utilizing data, sample client assessment procedures, and diagnostic and assessment measurements. The provision of sample forms for history-taking and the outreach and prevention materials in this section aid the professional in setting up educational situations. Section IV provides "Staff Development Resources," including an "Attitudes Towards Women Scale" and packaged training courses. Section V presents "Client Education Resources."

National Institute on Drug Abuse. *Youth at High Risk for Substance Abuse*. Washington, DC: Government Printing Office, 1987.

A technical review sponsored by a meeting of the National Institute on Drug Abuse, yielded papers and panel discussions on "Special Youth Populations, ---What Etiology Suggests About Prevention and Treatment Programming." This book provides papers and discussions focusing on four youth groups seen as high risk: juvenile delinquents, runaways, children in foster care programs, and children of substance abusers. The materials on children of substance abusers consider prevalence of drug problems, among them risk factors, (including genetic and environmental), and psychosocial issues. The book provides helpful references and reviews of research studies.

Northrup, Christiane. "The Patriarchal Myth and the Addictive System." In *Women's Bodies, Women's Wisdom*. New York: Bantam Books, 1995.

Noting that patriarchy is only one of many systems of social organization, Northrup considers its belief system concerning women. She finds, much like Anne Wilson Schaef, *Women's Reality* (Harper and Row, 1985), that patriarchy results in addiction, through demanding that women turn from their own hopes and dreams in deference to those of men and to the demands of their families. Northrup proceeds to list fundamental beliefs of the addictive system: that "Disease is the Enemy," that "Medical Science Is Omnipotent," and that "The Female Body Is Abnormal." She encourages women's reclamation of their own authority, through the power of naming and by healing pain and its consequences. This chapter contains helpful tables, one on the characteristics of the addictive system and one on the body as process, in distinction from the medical view. While this chapter does not treat individual process or substance addictions, it provides a framework for perceiving the subject, one applicable to individual addictions.

Rapping, Elayne. *The Culture of Recovery: Making Sense of the Self-Help Movement in Women's Lives.* Boston: Beacon Press, 1996.

The author bases this book on hundreds of hours of observing self-help meetings, among them Alcoholics Anonymous, Adult Children of Alcoholics, and Overeaters Anonymous. She also uses examples from interviews, books, and TV to present a major aspect of contemporary culture, the recovery movement. As she notices women joining the movement and seeking help for emotional and relational problems, Rapping also examines the recovery "industry," including treatment centers and talk shows. Rapping concludes, and rightfully, that the recovery phenomenon owes a good deal of its success to the insights and strategies of second wave feminism. What she finds unfortunate is that this same phenomenon seems to turn its back on the political message of the women's movement.

Schaef, Anne Wilson. *Women's Reality.* San Francisco: Harper and Row, 1985.

This second edition of the first of Schaef's book contains a new preface as well as including the preface to the first edition. Schaef began this book as a response to her realization that what she had learned formally had been useful in working with men but sometimes could be useless and sometimes harmful in working with women. She did soft research, setting aside a time of her life to learn about women. She, like Eileen Hoffman, *Our Health, Our Lives* (Bantam Books, 1995), dedicates her book to the women who have helped her learn, particularly clients. Clearly written, *Women's Reality* affords an opportunity for reflective comparison and contrast between what Schaef calls the "White Male System" and the "Emerging Female System." Chapter 4, "Stoppers," Chapter 6, "Paradox, Dualism, and Levels of Truth," and Chapter 7, "An Introduction to Female System Theology," are telling and concrete applications and instances of the more sweeping material in the book's other chapters. This work still provides the reader a chance to sigh with relief in recognizing what she has known for some time by seeing it

178 Women and Health

validated in the communication of other women. I have placed it in the chapter on addictions for two reasons: To keep the flow of Schaef's work intact for the reader and in recognition of the congruence between the addictive system and the White Male System, a congruence noted later in Schaef's writings.

Schaef, Anne Wilson. *Co-Dependence: Misunderstood-Mistreated.* San Franciso: Harper and Row, 1986.
At the time this book was written, codependence was a relatively new notion in the field of addictions. The term had been used to describe the condition of the spouse of the alcoholic. Schaef realized that in working on this concept, she might have an impact not only on chemical dependency but also on mental health, the women's movement, and family therapy. In fact, she did. A schema pointing to the connections among these fields, "The Addictive Process-A Generic, Systemic Disease," is delineated on page 23. This book presents a historical and developmental background of theories of codependence at the same time that it presents a theoretical conceptualization. Schaef suggests alternatives to the modes of treatment of codependency which were generally available at the time of this publication and considers the most important contribution of this book to be her postulate that codependency is a generic disease which she calls the addictive process.

Schaef, Anne Wilson. *When Society Becomes an Addict.* San Francisco: Harper & Row, 1987.
Breaking down barriers between the personal and the political, Schaef uses understandings of addiction behaviors in the individual to show the parallel patterns in public, social, and political groups. In pointing out, at the level of society, addictive patterns of living, the author draws from diverse disciplines and diverse insights. Her recognition that what she called "The White Male System" in her previous book, *Women's Reality* (Harper and Row, 1985), and what she calls "The Addictive System" in this book are one and the same is followed by a general introduction to

addiction. Making the discovery that larger systems (e.g., schools, churches, businesses, and governments) show the same characteristics, processes, problems, and outcomes as the individual addict, Schaef discusses the processes of the addictive system. In the final part of this book, the author discusses paradigm shifts as well as twelve-step programs, pointing toward ways in which these can be employed for systemic recovery.

Schaef, Anne Wilson, and Diane Fassel. *The Addictive Organization.* San Francisco: Harper and Row, 1988.

This sequel to Schaef's *When Society Becomes an Addict* (Harper and Row, 1987) deals with addictive systems in business, or similar group projects, and their dysfunctional behaviors. In it, Schaef and Fassel present four major modes of addictions in organizations: when the key person is an addict, when addictive behaviors learned elsewhere are brought to the organization, when the organization functions as an addictive substance, and when the organization as such is an addict. Unique to this book is its discussion of workaholism as a destructive addiction encouraged by society and appearing to profit the organization. What is uniquely helpful to those who have been socialized into believing they, as individuals, are the problem is that this book names, with readability and clarity, irrational traits which can inhere in an organization as such. For those seeking to understand or to recover from addiction, Schaef and Fassel's presentation provides reflective opportunity by naming qualities, behaviors, and consequences pertinent to any addiction.

Sher, Kenneth J. *Children of Alcoholics.* Chicago: University of Chicago Press, 1991.

This book attempts to build on earlier views concerning children of alcoholics by focusing on areas needing more research and further development. In particular, the author pays attention to issues of methodology in such research. While the author sees it as clear that alcohol abuse and dependence are prevalent phenomena and that a significant number of people are offspring of alcoholics, he is dissatisfied with considering these persons to be rather a homogeneous group. He finds most of the clinical literature to consider COAs (children of alcoholics) such and attempts to hone a category that he finds misleadingly broad. He also works at what he considers diagnostic imprecision and insufficient attention given to sources of heterogeneity in COAs. Since quite a bit is known about COAs and knowledge is growing rapidly, the author sifts and reviews what is known and not known and provides multiple frameworks for viewing the transmission of alcoholism and related problems through generations of families.

Stammer, M. Ellen, Ed.D. *Women and Alcohol: The Journey Back.* New York: Gardner Press, 1991.

Written originally as part of an Ed.D. dissertation, this book considers the cultural paths of women who are recovering from alcoholism. It is founded upon two assumptions: that it is possible to recover from alcoholism, a chronic, progressive, and possibly fatal disease, and that recovering women can reflect on their experience and share it with others. The author bases her considerations upon her work with 34 women participating in her study and sharing with her their lifeways. She compares lifeways to a river, meandering calmly at some times, deluging at others. The book is divided into three sections: "Growing Up," "Coping," and "Being Afraid." Within those parameters, Stammer discusses such issues as "Looking for Love," "Getting Alcohol Messages," "Feeling Worthless," "Becoming Aware," "Hitting Bottom," "Learning to Live," and "Accepting Self." This book can be read with enjoyment and profit by any interested woman or man. The data and dynamics are woven into the stories of the women involved in the study and are integrated into their expressions of cultural paths, or lifeways.

Steinem, Gloria. *Revolution from Within: A Book of Self-Esteem.* Boston: Little, Brown and Company, 1992.

For the twelve years previous to the idea for this book, Steinem had been addressing external barriers to women's equality. Recognizing that there are internal barriers and feeling that many of the books on self-esteem seemed incognizant of the structures which undermine women's self-worth, Steinem set about her research. She decided her book was for men too. While she had seen books directed at women's overempathy, she had not seen ones addressing men's underempathy, and she had seen books about low expectations for women in the public sphere but hardly any about low expectations for men in the private sphere. Explaining that in the course of writing her book she not only looked inward but also found a new prism through which to look outward, the author arrives at the need to takes leaps of imagination to address the issues of concern pertinent to the human community. She reverses that the adage the personal is political and points out that the political is personal. Particularly helpful to a number of readers are Chapter 3, "The Importance of Un-learning," and Chapter 4, "Re-learning."

Thoele, Sue Patton. *The Woman's Book of Courage*. Berkeley, CA: Conari Press, 1991.
Written by a woman with twenty years of experience as a therapeutic professional, this book compiles affirmations, meditations, and true stories which remind women of their own courage. The author notes that courage involves strength and willingness to do what the reader considers right even in the face of difficulty and fear. This book can be used as a guide to meditation, as a springboard for discussion, or as a common thread for an ongoing women's group. It encourages the reader to touch her own power and to claim those gifts in herself which are often seen by others but not experienced in her own self-understanding. It invites change in the reader, particularly that change which is new belief in self, with accompanying change in feelings and self-esteem.

Van Den Bergh, Nan, ed. *Feminist Perspectives on Addictions*. New York: Springer, 1991.

This book presents its topic in three divisions: "Gender Roles, Power, and Addictions," "Substance Dependencies," and "Process Dependencies." These divisions, by their very naming, point toward the major developments in the field of women and addictions during the 1970s and 1980s, that is, the larger cultural/political picture and the larger addictions picture beyond problems with individual substances. Chapter 7, "Double Jeopardy: Chemical Dependence and Codependence in Older Women," is read with great profit in conjunction with *Addiction Treatment for Older Adults*, Kathryn Graham (Haworth Press, 1995). Chapter 9, "Reclaiming Women's Bodies: A Feminist Perspective on Eating Disorders," is enhanced by reading it in tandem with Joan Jacobs Brumberg's *Fasting Girls* (Harvard University Press, 1988). The contributors to this book of essays are physicians, psychologists, sociologists, social workers, and certified addictions counselors, many of whom are well known for ongoing work in the field of addictions.

VanderVeen, Marilyn, John W. Stewart, and Susie Heritage. *Living Without Smoking: How to Survive When You're Ready to Quit.* Minneapolis, MN: Augsburg Fortress, 1989.

Written by a seminary student, a pastor, and a registered nurse, this book presents a successful smoking cessation program begun as a retreat for thirteen people from varying walks of life. Out of that experience grew a citywide ministry to help others quit smoking. The ministry was Christian-based, lay-led, inexpensive, and spiritually grounded. The authors of this book encourage its use as a personal tool for quitting, at the same time that they recommend belonging to a stop-smoking group. While the whole book provides help, there are some chapters of particular interest to would-be smoke-free persons. Chapter 2, "Why I Smoke," gives a checklist of reasons provided by the U.S. Department of Health and Human Services. Chapter 5, "How Can I Change," deals with principles and strategies of change. Chapter 8, "Goal Setting and Keeping a Journal," continues strategies by naming journaling as one and by instructing the reader in keeping a journal. Chapter 9, "Adjusting to

Loss," provides reflection on some of Elisabeth Kubler-Ross's work showing its implications for the loss experienced in giving up smoking. Chapter 10, "How to Handle Stress-Without Smoking," provides a functional description of stress and strategies for meeting it without cigarettes.

Vourakis, Christine. "Drug Abuse Problems Among Women." In Catherine Ingram Fogel and Nancy Fugate Woods, eds., *Women's Health Care: A Comprehensive Handbook.* Thousand Oaks, CA: Sage Publications, 1995.

Chapter 22, "Drug Abuse Problems Among Women," presents a definition of terms combined with an enlightening historical perspective. It cites the prevalence of drug abuse among women, offering specific considerations concerning alcohol and other drugs. Listing the effects of alcohol and other drugs during pregnancy, it presents the issues around criminal punishment of drug-dependent pregnant women. The selected issues for intervention include not only the effects of drugs on women's bodies generally but also specific concerns with regard to gender roles and chemical dependency, depression and chemically dependent women, and AIDS. The chapter ends with a discussion of treatment and prevention issues. The references at the end of this chapter provide the reader an avenue of further exploration.

Wallen, Jaqueline, Ph.D. *Addiction in Human Development: Developmental Perspectives on Addiction and Recovery.* New York: The Haworth Press, 1993.

In considering addiction as a health issue and in considering wellness across the lifespan, the developmental model of this work offers helpful insight. Noting that a developmental perspective deals with how individuals change and grow throughout life, the author uses the concepts of developmental stages and unresolved developmental tasks to provide examples of developmental theory. This book for substance abuse and mental health professionals is so clearly and straightforwardly written that it can also be read with profit and enjoyment by other interested persons. In discussing "Developmental Issues in Recovery," Wallen presents Erikson's stages of development as well as considerations on spiritual development. She presents stages of change through cognitive-developmental lenses in Chapter 2, "Recovery as a Developmental Process," and considers delayed stress reactions and responses as these pertain to childhood trauma in Chapter 3, "Developmental Trauma and Recovery." Treating "Family Recovery as a Developmental Process" in Chapter 4, Wallen discusses "The Intergenerational Transmission of Addiction and Recovery" in Chapter 5. Like Sharon Wegschieder's approach in *Another Chance* (Science and Behavior Books, 1981), Wallen puts forth personal and professional considerations for the practitioner in the field in Chapter 6, "Developmental Issues for the Professional." The three appendices of this book are enriching as well as practical reading: Appendix A, "Short Michigan Alcoholism Screening Test," Appendix B "Piaget's Cognitive-Developmental Stages," and Appendix C, "Moral Development." While this book is generally helpful, it pays scant to no attention to women's developmental issues per se and mentions once, in passing, that some have questioned the universality of Kohlberg's stages of moral development.

Wegschieder, Sharon. *Another Chance: Hope and Health for the Alcoholic Family.* Palo Alto, CA: Science and Behavior Books, 1981. One of the earlier and more widely read books on alcoholism and the family, this work has a foreword by Virginia Satin and another by Kenneth Williams. With extensive clinical experience as well as personal experience with the pain and issues of families experiencing the dysfunction of alcohol addiction, Wegschieder raises to view the loneliness, fear, shame, guilt , hurt, and courage of families breaking their secret and moving toward a new health. Introducing a model of understanding based upon family scenario roles, the author presents the alcohol Dependent as well as the supporting cast of the Enabler, the

Hero, the Scapegoat, the Lost Child, and the Mascot. These heuristic devices help the reader to see the dynamics the family uses to try to regain some equilibrium when family balance is disrupted by addictive disease. Wegschieder offers hope by pointing out that intervention and wellness are possible. She offers this hope not only through the power of naming and understanding the situation but also by presenting treatment dynamics for recovery. These include primary care, aftercare, self-help groups, and support. Breakthrough contributions of this book were its model for describing the members of the family cast and its taking seriously the needs of each and the needs of the whole in a holistic manner. Wegschieder's "Whole Person Wheel" is a helpful and manageable diagram which can aid anyone in tending to whole health. Appendix A, "Exercises for Healthier Families," and Appendix B, " The Whole Person Inventory," provide the reader, whether professional or nonprofessional, ways of tending to ongoing wholeness.

Whitfield, Charles L. *A Gift to Myself: A Personal Workbook and Guide to Healing the Child Within.* Deerfield Beach, FL: Health Communications, 1990.

This publication, which can be used as an accompanying workbook for Whitfield's *Healing the Child Within* (Health Communications, 1987), offers exercises constructed to assist adult children in recovering from the consequences of developing in a dysfunctional family (e.g., an alcoholic one). Designed for rediscovering the inner self, these exercises elicit the identification of needs and feelings and foster the grieving and resolution of losses related to past traumas. The author, in proffering the exercises, assists the reader in working through the issues and the dynamics of codependence. Describing stages of recovery, the book provides strategies in choosing a support group or a therapist for the ACOA (adult child of an alcoholic) seeking further help. A sample form for exploring problems in one's family of origin and a family drinking survey are included in the appendices.

Whitfield, Charles L. *Healing the Child Within: Discovery and Recovery for Adult Children of Dysfunctional Families.* Deerfield Beach, FL: Health Communications, 1987.

This work consider the ways in which a dysfunctional family situation elicits the development of a codependent self and creates problems with free expression of feelings. Offering guidelines to help the reader in learning to accept and deal with repressed emotions, the book provides charts, tables, and questionnaires as aids for self-assessment. Written for adults who experienced acute or prolonged childhood traumas (e.g., parental alcoholism, physical or sexual abuse), the book concentrates on recovering the child within, that is inner self, with feelings, desires, creativity, and spontaneity. In rediscovering the inner self, the reader is offered ways for restoring and nurturing that inner child.

Woititz, Janet Geringer, Ed.D. *Adult Children of Alcoholics.* Pompano Beach, FL: Health Communications, 1983.

One of the earlier works attending specifically to adult children of alcoholics (ACOA) rather than calling them alcoholics or spouses of alcoholics, this book acknowledges the full measure of ACOA's exposure to alcoholism and identifies applicable characteristics further. It pays specific attention to the children living in alcoholic homes, discussing how poor self-image displays itself and offering suggestions regarding ways to change, if change is desirable. Woititz, having worked with groups of adult children of alcoholics, provides an in-depth look at their thoughts, feelings, attitudes, and reactions, as well as the pervasively powerful influence of alcohol in their lives. She comes to generalizations, occurring in one guise or another, and finds these generalizations worthy of attention, listing them in thirteen statements. She uses these statements as a skeleton for raising examination, discussion, insight, suggestions, and clarity as her book proceeds.

Woititz, Janet Geringer, Ed.D. *Struggle for Intimacy.* Pompano Beach, FL: Health Communications, 1985.

Dedicated to adult children of alcoholics, this book treats the complex issue of intimacy, particularly in that population. Beginning with considerations on whom one picks for a lover, Woititz points out the dysfunctional opposite messages which can drive the selection. That directs her to consider the description of a healthy relationship and to discuss relationship issues. This latter she does by considering myths held by ACOAs (adult children of alcoholics) and by making responses to them. Her chapter on issues of sexuality deals with those issues in terms of heterosexual as well as homosexual couples. It is followed by a discussion of what may be expected and how to work at a relationship if one loves a child of an alcoholic. The author's final chapter, "Getting It All Together," provides a review of some of the characteristics of ACOAs with advice on approaches to relational growth. This book is well read in tandem with Woititz's *Adult Children of Alcoholics* (Health Communications, 1983) and is a further drawing out of the implications of her discoveries on that topic.

Youcha, Geraldine. *A Dangerous Pleasure.* New York: Hawthorn Books, 1978.

A magazine and newspaper columnist, Youcha sees herself as one who reports on the social scene. Her chapter "Superior but Not Equal" deals with the double bind of women experiencing alcoholism, what Gerda Lerner has pointed out to be the cult of the lady. That double standard has, until recently, kept large numbers of women from receiving the help necessary to recover. Youcha's work presents in very readable language, and early in the research on women and alcoholism, the differences between men and women with regard to alcohol and alcohol problems. She alludes to the danger of synergistic reactions to combinations of other drugs and alcohol. She mentions data pertinent to fetal alcohol syndrome. Helpful to the reader are a checklist for those who question whether they have a drinking problem and "A Guide to Sensible Drinking."

Zimberg, Sheldon, John Wallace, and Sheila B. Blume, eds. *Practical Approaches to Alcoholism Psychotherapy*. New York: Plenum Press, 1985. The focus on prevention as well as on practical responses to alcoholism have made this book a contribution to the field of addictions therapy. This second edition differs from the first (1978) in that it not only updates previous material but also provides new chapters on differential diagnosis, biological factors in alcoholism, treatment for children of alcoholics, couples therapy, diagnosis and treatment of sexual dysfunctions in alcoholics, the use of intervention techniques, and the employment of social network therapy. Chapter 14, "The Psychotherapy of Alcoholic Women," is limited in that it is based upon work done primarily with city and suburban women. It does, however, attempt to sift between male and female experiences of alcoholism, and it does posit considerable intragroup differences among women.

AUTHOR INDEX

Isasi-Diaz, Ada Maria, 27

Jacobson, Jodi, 140
Jarvik, Lissy, M.D., Ph.D., and Gary Small,
    M.D., 141
Johnson, Elizabeth A., 27
Johnson, Karen, M.D., and Tom Ferguson,
    M.D., 119
Jordan, Judith V., Alexandra G. Kaplan,
    Jean Baker Miller, Irene P. Striver, and
    Janet L. Surrey, 28

Kahn, Ada P., and Linda Hughes Holt,
    M.D., 120
Kaledin, Eugenia, 28
Kaminer, Wendy, 142
Kessler-Harris, Alice, 29
Ketcham, Katherine, and Ginny L.
    Gustafson, 171
King, Pat, 172
Kirkpatrick, Jean, Ph.D., 172
Klein, Anne Carolyn, 173
Kosof, Anna, 66
Kramarae, Chris, and Dale Spender, 29
Kurth, Ann, 66
Kurtz, Ron, 121

Larrington, Carolyne, 30
Learn, Cheryl Demerath, 92
Leavitt, Judith W., 30
Leeson, Joyce, and Judith Gray, 93
Legato, Marianne, M.D., and Carol Colman,
    66
Leonard, Ann, 67
Lerner, Gerda, 31
Lerner, Rokelle, 174
Levin, Beatrice, 93
Levine, Susan, 142
Lewis, Judith A., and Judith Bernstein, 94
Lopate, Carol, 95
Lorber, Judith, 95
Lowe. Marian, and Ruth Hubbard, 32
Luker, Kristin, 68
Lustbader, Wendy, and Nancy R. Hooyman,
    143
Lutter, Judy Mahle, and Lynn Jaffee, 121

McClain, Carol Shepherd, 96
McFague, Sallie, 32, 174
McGoon, Michael D., 68
McKenny, Gerald P., and Jonathan R.
    Sande, 33

McLeod, Eileen, 69
Mahowald, Mary Briody, 69
Matteo, Sherri, 70
Matthews, Glenna, 33
Melosh, Barbara, 34, 96, 97, 144
Miller, Dorothy C., 144
Miller, Jean Baker, 35
Miller, Norman S., 174
Miner, Valerie, and Helen E. Longino, 70
Mirsky, Judith, 71
Morantz-Sanchez, Regina Markell, 97
Morawski, Jill G., 35
Muller, Charlotte F., 71
Myers, Henry, 145

National Institute on Alcohol Abuse and
    Alcoholism, 175
National Institute on Drug Abuse, 176
Nechas, Eileen, and Denise Foley, 72
Neuger, Christie Cozad, 98
Nicarthy, Ginny, Naomi Gottlieb, and
    Sandra Hoffman, 122
Norsigian, Judy, 146
Northrup, Christiane, M.D., 72, 98, 99
Numbers, Ronald L., and Darrel W.
    Amundsen, 35

Oakley, Ann, 73

Payne, Elizabeth Anne, 146
Plant, Judith, 36
Plaskow, Judith, 36

Quaid, Maeve, 147

Raffo, Susan, 147
Rapping, Elayne, 177
Raymond, Janice, 37
Rosser, Sue, 37
Rothman, Barbara, 38
Royston, Erica, and Sue Armstrong, 74

Samuelson, Michael H., 122
Schaef, Anne Wilson, 177-179
Schaef, Anne Wilson, and Diane Fassel, 179
Schaefer, Charles E., Ph.D., and Theresa
    DiGeronimo, M.Ed., 123
Scott, Niki, 148
Scully, Diana, 123
Sen, Gita, Adrienne Germain, and C. Chen,
    148
Sheehy, Gail, 124, 125

TITLE INDEX

193

SUBJECT INDEX

abortion, 19, 21, 68-70, 149, 150
abuse, 14, 33, 43, 47, 54, 59, 66, 79, 86, 87,
    115-117, 119, 120, 122, 123, 132, 133,
    160-162, 165, 168, 170-172, 175, 176,
    180, 183, 186
academics, 19, 56, 108, 116
activism, 8, 36, 46, 56, 66, 100, 147
activists, 19, 20, 44, 68, 78, 81, 148
addictions, 88, 107, 155, 156, 161, 163,
    164, 168, 174-176, 178, 179, 181, 182,
    188
adolescents, 63
African American, 7, 29, 42, 44, 101, 105,
    153 (see also Black women).
AIDS, 38, 46, 47, 49, 62, 66, 70-72, 113,
    121, 123, 126, 127, 143, 183
alcoholic, 123, 158, 159, 165-167, 169,
    173, 175, 178, 184-188
androcentric, 33, 37, 38, 56, 157
anthropology, 21, 22, 96, 101, 125
Asia, 92, 112
Asian(s), 44, 112
attitudes, 6, 11, 12, 15, 19, 34, 47, 58, 62,
    64, 65, 68, 90, 94, 110, 119, 123, 124,
    135, 142, 153, 174, 186

backlash, 16, 17
battered women, 56, 59, 66, 76, 88, 156
beliefs, 18, 64, 65, 67, 101, 106, 132-134,
    171, 176
biological determinism, 18
biology, 26, 48, 67, 164, 175
Black women, 19, 72, 78, 82, 91, 92, 105
    (see also African American).
body, 2, 11, 13, 19, 20, 23, 24, 32, 43, 45,
    48, 50, 51, 54, 55, 67, 74, 77, 79, 81, 84,
    89, 99, 101, 106, 108-111, 113, 116,
    117, 121, 122, 127, 138, 149, 150, 155,
    161, 165, 171, 174, 176
Buddhism, 22, 23, 121, 173

CAD, 117
Canadian(s), 8, 12, 55, 64, 83, 84, 94
cardiac, 2, 44, 67

childbearing, 20, 30, 31, 74, 113, 114, 133,
    174
Chinese, 37
Christianity, 8, 12, 14, 21-23, 27, 86
clinical judgments, 10
codependent, 109, 158, 186
compassion, 24, 53, 103, 121, 173
competition, 11, 20, 70, 71
conflict, 20, 31, 35, 83, 97, 127, 144
covenant, 33, 95
crone, 13, 23, 24, 129
culture, 6, 11, 13, 17, 22, 27, 32, 34, 39, 58,
    83, 96, 97, 140, 144, 164, 165, 177

disempowerment, 33
diversity, 8, 19, 27, 37, 46, 53, 54, 63, 69,
    78, 96, 105, 110, 113, 119, 121, 146,
    149

eating disorders, 28, 43, 88, 118, 120, 122,
    182
ecofeminism, 21, 36
ecology, 14, 15, 68
economic dependence, 20
economy, 8, 10, 29, 134, 135, 137-139,
    151, 152
education, 3, 9, 11, 26, 29, 37, 48, 52, 64,
    67, 68, 70, 80, 81, 83, 87, 93, 98,
    107-109, 111, 114, 115, 126, 128, 129,
    131, 133, 150, 164, 175
egalitarian, 10, 69
elder, 81, 158
embodiment, 32
empowerment, 33, 90, 101, 109, 128, 147,
    148
environment, 36, 116, 121, 134, 149, 153
epistemologies, 1, 4, 21, 38, 80, 107
equality, 16, 17, 76, 126, 135, 181
ethics, 7, 14, 20, 25, 33, 38, 39, 72, 80, 86,
    98, 114, 115, 149
exercise, 40, 41, 73, 99, 109, 113, 114, 122,

family roles, 29, 61
femininity, 11, 23, 52, 53

199

ABOUT THE AUTHOR

Dr. Frances R. Belmonte, Ph.D., icadc is a member of the Graduate Faculty, Loyola University Chicago and Associate Professor at its Institute of Pastoral Studies. A systematic and pastoral theologian with expertise in spirituality, imagination, and feminist concerns, Dr. Belmonte also teaches Medical Humanities to fourth year medical students at Loyola's Stritch School of Medicine. She has been involved in co-facilitating Health Care Ministries Integration Seminar for nursing, theology and seminary students in the Chicago area. Resident Theologian for the Bishop and people of the Catholic Diocese of Memphis for a six year period, she also served as page editor and weekly columnist for its diocesan newspaper. Dr. Belmonte holds an internationally reciprocal senior clinical certification in Substance Abuse Counseling.